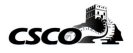

中国临床肿瘤学会（CSCO）
造血干细胞移植治疗血液系统疾病指南
2023

GUIDELINES OF CHINESE SOCIETY OF CLINICAL ONCOLOGY (CSCO)
HSCT FOR HEMATOLOGICAL DISEASES

中国临床肿瘤学会指南工作委员会　组织编写

人民卫生出版社
·北京·

版权所有，侵权必究！

图书在版编目（CIP）数据

中国临床肿瘤学会（CSCO）造血干细胞移植治疗血液系统疾病指南.2023/中国临床肿瘤学会指南工作委员会组织编写.—北京：人民卫生出版社，2023.4

ISBN 978-7-117-34673-3

Ⅰ.①中⋯　Ⅱ.①中⋯　Ⅲ.①造血干细胞—干细胞移植—指南　Ⅳ.①R550.5-62

中国国家版本馆 CIP 数据核字（2023）第 050780 号

人卫智网	www.ipmph.com	医学教育、学术、考试、健康，购书智慧智能综合服务平台
人卫官网	www.pmph.com	人卫官方资讯发布平台

中国临床肿瘤学会（CSCO）造血干细胞移植治疗血液系统疾病指南 2023
Zhongguo Linchuang Zhongliu Xuehui（CSCO）Zaoxue Ganxibao Yizhi Zhiliao Xueye Xitong Jibing Zhinan 2023

组织编写：中国临床肿瘤学会指南工作委员会
出版发行：人民卫生出版社（中继线 010-59780011）
地　　址：北京市朝阳区潘家园南里 19 号
邮　　编：100021
E - mail：pmph @ pmph.com
购书热线：010-59787592　010-59787584　010-65264830
印　　刷：三河市宏达印刷有限公司（胜利）
打击盗版举报电话：010-59787491　E-mail：WQ @ pmph.com
质量问题联系电话：010-59787234　E-mail：zhiliang @ pmph.com
数字融合服务电话：4001118166　　E-mail：zengzhi @ pmph.com

经　　销：新华书店
开　　本：787×1092　1/32　印张：7.5
字　　数：201 千字
版　　次：2023 年 4 月第 1 版
印　　次：2023 年 4 月第 1 次印刷
标准书号：ISBN 978-7-117-34673-3
定　　价：62.00 元

中国临床肿瘤学会指南工作委员会

组　长　徐瑞华　　李　进

副组长　（以姓氏汉语拼音为序）

　　　　程　颖　　樊　嘉　　郭　军　　赫　捷　　江泽飞
　　　　梁　军　　梁后杰　　马　军　　秦叔逵　　王　洁
　　　　吴令英　　吴一龙　　殷咏梅　　于金明　　朱　军

中国临床肿瘤学会（CSCO）
造血干细胞移植治疗血液系统疾病指南

2023

组　　　长	黄晓军　吴德沛　马　军	
副 组 长	刘启发　许兰平	
秘 书 组	刘代红　张　曦　贡铁军	

专家组成员（以姓氏汉语拼音为序）（* 为执笔人）

陈文明*　　首都医科大学附属北京朝阳医院
陈育红*　　北京大学人民医院
窦立萍　　中国人民解放军总医院第五医学中心
范志平*　　南方医科大学南方医院
贡铁军　　哈尔滨血液病肿瘤研究所
胡　炯*　　上海交通大学医学院附属瑞金医院
黄晓军*　　北京大学人民医院
姜尔烈　　中国医学科学院血液病医院
刘代红*　　中国人民解放军总医院第五医学中心

刘启发*	南方医科大学南方医院
马　军	哈尔滨血液病肿瘤研究所
莫晓冬*	北京大学人民医院
唐晓文*	苏州大学附属第一医院
王　昱*	北京大学人民医院
王小沛*	北京大学肿瘤医院
王志国	哈尔滨血液病肿瘤研究所
吴德沛*	苏州大学附属第一医院
许兰平*	北京大学人民医院
张　曦*	中国人民解放军陆军军医大学第二附属医院（新桥医院）
张圆圆*	北京大学人民医院

前言

基于循证医学证据、兼顾诊疗产品的可及性、吸收精准医学新进展，制定中国常见肿瘤的诊断和治疗指南，是中国临床肿瘤学会（CSCO）的基本任务之一。近年来，临床诊疗指南的制定出现新的趋向，即基于诊疗资源的可及性，这尤其适合于发展中国家，以及地区差异性显著的国家和地区。中国是幅员辽阔、地区经济和学术发展不平衡的发展中国家，CSCO指南需要兼顾地区发展差异、药物和诊疗手段的可及性及肿瘤治疗的社会价值三个方面。因此，CSCO指南的制定，要求每一个临床问题的诊疗意见根据循证医学证据和专家共识度形成证据类别，同时结合产品的可及性和效价比形成推荐等级。证据类别高、可及性好的方案，作为Ⅰ级推荐；证据类别较高、专家共识度稍低，或可及性较差的方案，作为Ⅱ级推荐；临床实用，但证据类别不高的，作为Ⅲ级推荐。CSCO指南主要基于国内外临床研究成果和CSCO专家意见，确定推荐等级，以便于大家在临床实践中参考使用。CSCO指南工作委员会相信，基于证据、兼顾可及、结合意见的指南，更适合我国的临床实际。我们期待得到大家宝贵的反馈意见，并将在指南更新时认真考虑、积极采纳合理建议，保持CSCO指南的科学性、公正性和时效性。

中国临床肿瘤学会指南工作委员会

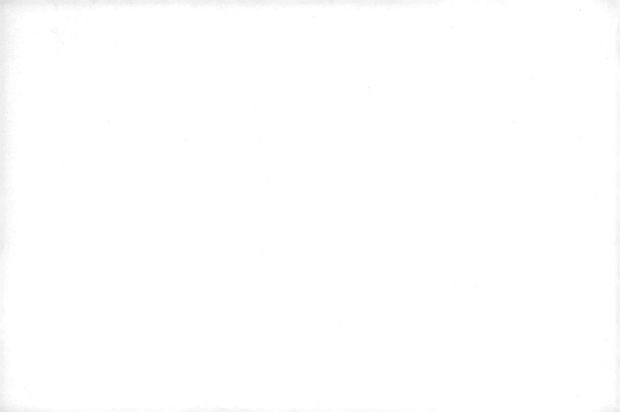

目录

CSCO 诊疗指南证据类别 • 1
CSCO 诊疗指南推荐等级 • 2
总则 • 3
异基因造血干细胞移植 • 7

  1 异基因造血干细胞移植治疗血液系统疾病的适应证及移植时机 • 8
      1.1 急性髓性白血病（≤65 岁） • 8
      1.2 急性淋巴细胞白血病（≤65 岁） • 12
      1.3 慢性髓性白血病（≤65 岁） • 16
      1.4 骨髓增生异常综合征（≤65 岁） • 18
      1.5 多发性骨髓瘤 • 19
      1.6 淋巴瘤 • 20
      1.7 重型再生障碍性贫血（≤60 岁） • 25
  2 异基因造血干细胞移植治疗血液系统疾病的供者选择 • 31
      2.1 供者来源选择 • 31
      2.2 非体外去除 T 细胞单倍型相合供者选择 • 33
      2.3 非血缘志愿者供者选择 • 37
      2.4 非血缘脐带血供者选择 • 40

目录

3 异基因造血干细胞移植前患者及供者评估 • 47
    3.1 患者评估 • 47
    3.2 供者移植前评估 • 50

4 异基因造血干细胞移植预处理方案 • 52
    4.1 标准清髓性（MAC）预处理 • 52
    4.2 减低毒性（RTC）、降低强度（RIC）或非清髓（NMA）预处理 • 54
    4.3 增强预处理和强化疗序贯移植预处理 • 57
    4.4 重度再生障碍性贫血（SAA）移植预处理 • 59

5 异基因造血干细胞移植供者动员、细胞采集及回输 • 64

6 异基因造血干细胞移植后急性移植物抗宿主病的预防、诊断及治疗 • 69
    6.1 急性移植物抗宿主病预防药物推荐 • 69
    6.2 急性移植物抗宿主病预防药物用药方法推荐 • 72
    6.3 急性移植物抗宿主病诊断及分度标准 • 75
    6.4 急性移植物抗宿主病治疗药物推荐 • 77

7 异基因造血干细胞移植慢性移植物抗宿主病的预防、诊断及治疗 • 84
    7.1 慢性移植物抗宿主病的预防 • 84
    7.2 慢性移植物抗宿主病的诊断 • 87

- 7.3 慢性移植物抗宿主病的一线治疗 • 89
- 7.4 慢性移植物抗宿主病的二线治疗 • 90

8 **异基因造血干细胞移植过程中真菌感染的预防及治疗** • 101
- 8.1 真菌感染的预防 • 101
- 8.2 真菌感染的治疗 • 102

9 **异基因造血干细胞移植过程中病毒感染的检测、预防及治疗** • 109
- 9.1 异基因造血干细胞移植中乙型病毒性肝炎管理 • 109
- 9.2 造血干细胞移植中巨细胞病毒感染管理 • 113
- 9.3 异基因造血干细胞移植后 EB 病毒感染的管理 • 120

10 **异基因造血干细胞移植后白血病/骨髓增生异常综合征复发的监测、预防、治疗** • 130
- 10.1 移植后复发的监测 • 130
- 10.2 移植后复发的预防 • 136
- 10.3 移植后复发的抢先治疗 • 143
- 10.4 移植后复发的治疗 • 148

11 **异基因造血干细胞移植后随访** • 158

自体造血干细胞移植 • 161

1 适应证 • 162

目录

    1.1 淋巴瘤自体移植适应证 • 162

    1.2 多发性骨髓瘤自体造血干细胞移植适应证 • 167

2 动员方案 • 169

    2.1 干细胞动员方案与冻存 • 169

    2.2 造血干细胞采集 • 170

3 临床应用 • 172

    3.1 自体造血干细胞移植治疗多发性骨髓瘤 • 172

    3.2 自体造血干细胞移植治疗淋巴瘤 • 178

附录 • 191

附录 1 AML（非 APL）危险分层标准 • 192

附录 2 CML 在 TKI 治疗后的疗效反应 • 193

附录 3 MDS 的国际预后积分系统（IPSS） • 194

附录 4 MDS 修订国际预后积分系统（IPSS-R） • 195

附录 5 MDS 的 WHO 分型预后积分系统（WPSS） • 196

附录 6 异基因造血干细胞移植前患者应符合的条件 • 197

附录 7 造血干细胞移植合并症指数（HSCT-CI） • 198

附录 8 改良的急性 GVHD Glucksberg 分级 • 201

附录 9　IBMTR 的急性 GVHD 严重度指数　• 203
附录 10　MAGIC 分级标准（aGVHD 国际联盟 GVHD 分度）　• 204
附录 11　慢性移植物抗宿主病的临床征象　• 206
附录 12　慢性移植物抗宿主病（cGVHD）分级评分系统　• 208
附录 13　HSCT 患者 HBV 感染 / 再激活定义　• 212
附录 14　乙肝血清免疫学标志物检测内容和临床意义　• 213
附录 15　CMV 感染 / 再激活的诊断　• 214
附录 16　CMV 感染 / 再激活的危险因素　• 217
附录 17　CMV 感染治疗的常用药物及用法　• 218
附录 18　EBV 疾病的诊断　• 219
附录 19　特异性器官的长期随访评估　• 220

CSCO 诊疗指南证据类别

证据特征			CSCO 专家共识度
类别	水平	来源	
1A	高	严谨的 meta 分析、大型随机对照研究	一致共识 (支持意见 ≥ 80%)
1B	高	严谨的 meta 分析、大型随机对照研究	基本一致共识 (支持意见 60% ~ <80%)
2A	稍低	一般质量的 meta 分析、小型随机对照研究、设计良好的大型回顾性研究、病例-对照研究	一致共识 (支持意见 ≥ 80%)
2B	稍低	一般质量的 meta 分析、小型随机对照研究、设计良好的大型回顾性研究、病例-对照研究	基本一致共识 (支持意见 60% ~ <80%)
3	低	非对照的单臂临床研究、病例报告、专家观点	无共识,且争议大 (支持意见 <60%)

CSCO 诊疗指南推荐等级

推荐等级	标准
Ⅰ级推荐	**1A 类证据和部分 2A 类证据** CSCO 指南将 1A 类证据，以及部分专家共识度高且在中国可及性好的 2A 类证据，作为Ⅰ级推荐。具体为：适应证明确、可及性好、肿瘤治疗价值稳定，纳入《国家基本医疗保险、工伤保险和生育保险药品目录》的诊治措施
Ⅱ级推荐	**1B 类证据和部分 2A 类证据** CSCO 指南将 1B 类证据，以及部分在中国可及性欠佳，但专家共识度较高的 2A 类证据，作为Ⅱ级推荐。具体为：国内外随机对照研究，提供高级别证据，但可及性差或者效价比不高；对于临床获益明显但价格较贵的措施，考虑患者可能获益，也可作为Ⅱ级推荐
Ⅲ级推荐	**2B 类证据和 3 类证据** 对于某些临床上习惯使用，或有探索价值的诊治措施，虽然循证医学证据相对不足，但专家组意见认为可以接受的，作为Ⅲ级推荐

总则

异基因造血干细胞移植（allo-HSCT）是根治白血病、骨髓增生异常综合征（myelodysplastic syndrome，MDS）、多发性骨髓瘤（multiple myoloma，MM）、非霍奇金淋巴瘤（non Hodgkin lymphoma，NHL）和重症再生障碍性贫血（SAA）的有效手段，随着单倍型相合造血干细胞移植（haplo-HSCT）"北京方案"的建立及在中国广泛地应用，allo-HSCT进入了"人人都有供者的时代"，由此我国的HSCT病例数量快速增长[1-3]。北京方案最早用于白血病的治疗，近年来在SAA、MM和NHL上也获得了突破性进展，haplo-HSCT治疗SAA获得了和同胞全相合移植相似的疗效。国际上以人类白细胞抗原（human leukocyte antigen，HLA）配型相合同胞供者和非血缘供者allo-HSCT为主要证据支撑的移植指南，已经不能满足我国的临床需求，因此，由中国临床肿瘤学会（CSCO）组织，编写了《异基因造血干细胞移植治疗白血病和MDS指南2021版》，该指南参考了多个国际指南及中国异基因造血干细胞移植专家共识[4-6]，纳入了中国的临床研究成果。2022年对2021版指南的部分内容进行了更新并增加了SAA/vSAA的内容更名为《异基因造血干细胞移植治疗血液系统疾病指南2022版》，2023年在内容更新的基础上增加了异基因HSCT和自体HSCT治疗MM和NHL的内容。本指南将继续随着移植技术的进步和研究结果的丰富而更新。

参考文献

[1] XU LP, WU DP, HAN MZ, et al. A review of hematopoietic cell transplantation in China: Data and trends during 2008-2016. Bone Marrow Transplant, 2017, 52 (11): 1512-1518.

[2] XU LP, LU DP, WU DP, et al. Hematopoietic stem cell transplantation activity in China 2020-2021 during the SARS-

CoV-2 pandemic: A report from the Chinese Blood and Marrow Transplantation Registry Group. Transplant Cell Ther, 2023, 29 (2): 136e1-136e7.
[3] CHANG YJ, PEI XY, HUANG XJ. Haematopoietic stem-cell transplantation in China in the era of targeted therapies: Current advances, challenges, and future directions. Lancet Haematol, 2022, 9 (12): e919-e929.
[4] ZHANG XH, CHEN J, HAN MZ, et al. The consensus from The Chinese Society of Hematology on indications, conditioning regimens and donor selection for allogeneic hematopoietic stem cell transplantation: 2021 update. J Hematol Oncol, 2021, 14 (1): 145.
[5] 中华医学会血液学分会干细胞应用学组. 中国异基因造血干细胞移植治疗血液系统疾病专家共识(Ⅲ): 急性移植物抗宿主病(2020年版). 中华血液学杂志, 2020, 41 (7): 529-536.
[6] WANG Y, CHEN H, CHEN J, et al. The consensus on the monitoring, treatment, and prevention of leukemia relapse after allogeneic hematopoietic stem cell transplantation in China. Cancer Lett, 2018, 438: 63-75.

异基因造血干细胞移植

1 异基因造血干细胞移植治疗血液系统疾病的适应证及移植时机

1.1 急性髓性白血病（≤65 岁）

疾病分类	疾病状态分层	I 级推荐	II 级推荐	III 级推荐
APL	CR1			巩固治疗中 MRD 未转阴或巩固治疗结束后分子学复发后经治疗骨髓 PML-RARa 不能持续阴性的患者（3 类）
	≥CR2			1. 血液学复发后经治疗达 HCR 但骨髓 PML-RARaMRD 阳性（3 类） 2. ≥CR2 患者分子学复发经治疗骨髓 PPML-RARa 不能持续转阴的患者（3 类）
	复发/难治患者			Allo-HSCT，个性化移植方案（3 类）

急性髓性白血病（≤65 岁）（续）

疾病分类	疾病状态分层	I 级推荐	II 级推荐	III 级推荐
AML (Non-APL)	CR1	ELN/NCCN 指南危险度分层为高危的患者（2A 类）tAML-AML、MRC-AML 或具有前驱 MDS/CMML 的 AML（2A 类）ELN/NCCN 指南危险度分层为低危，在 MRD 指导下选择出对早期化疗分子学反应差的患者（2A 类）	ELN/NCCN 指南危险度分层中危的患者 CR1 移植（2A 类）	
	≥CR2	Allo-HSCT（2A 类）		
	复发/难治	Allo-HSCT，移植前减瘤或预处理方案加强（2A 类）		

【注释】

AML 预后分层标准见附录 1。

当不移植的预期复发率达 35%~40% 以上应该考虑在第一次缓解期进行异基因造血干细胞移植。欧洲白血病网（European Leukmia Net，ELN）或美国国立综合癌症网络（National Comprehensive Cancer Network，NCCN）分层为中高危的急性髓性白血病（AML）患者第一次缓解期（CR1）移植，在回顾性病例对照研究、前瞻性研究中均获支持[1-4]。在一项针对中危 AML 前瞻性队列研究中，患者经诱导 1~2 个疗程后达 CR1，4 个月仍在 CR1 期的患者 147 例，其中 69 例继续化疗，78 例接受单倍体造血干细胞移植，移植组 3 年无病生存率（LFS）和存活率（OS）均优于化疗组（74.3% vs. 47.3%；80.8% vs. 53.5%），多因素分析显示治疗方式是影响 LFS、OS 和复发的危险因素[4]。ELN 或 NCCN 分层为低危非急性早幼粒细胞白血病（non-APL）-AML 患者，基于化疗早期微小残留病（MRD）动态变化筛选出高危患者，这些患者在 CR1 期接受 allo-HSCT 获益[5-9]。每种白血病 MRD 的变化规律与预后的关系均有研究。一项多中心 AML05 前瞻性研究分析了 116 例 t（8；21）AML 患者的资料，将 RUNX1-RUNX1 AML 患者巩固强化 2 个疗程后 RUNX1-RUNX1 转录本水平较基线下降 <3 个对数级或 6 个月内失去 MMR 者定义为复发高危患者，结果显示，高危患者从移植获益，而非高危患者化疗效果预后更佳[5]。在儿童 t（8；21）AML 中将高危定义为巩固 2 个疗程后 RUNX1-RUNX1 转录本水平 >0.05%，也得到类似结论[6]。另一项回顾性研究分析了 58 例 CBFB-MYH11（+）AML，25 例移植，33 例化疗，结果发现 2 次巩固化疗后 CBFB-MYH11/ABL 在任何时间曾 >0.1% 患者为复发高危组，这些高危患者获益于移植（LFS 移植组 84.6%，化疗组 31.4%，$P<0.001$）[7]。一项队

列研究分析 124 例新诊断的 CEBPA^{bi+} AML 患者，巩固 2 个疗程后持续 MRD 阳性和任何时间点失去 MRD 阴性状态为高危患者，这些患者获益于异基因移植（3 年累计复发率移植组 0，化疗组 52.8%；$P=0.006$；3 年 LFS 移植组 88.9%，化疗组 47.2%；$P=0.027$）[8]。一项针对 NPM1 突变患者的回顾性研究发现 2 次巩固治疗 MRD 高水平（*NPM1* 突变转录本水平下降<3 个对数级）是影响化疗后 DFS 的危险因素，具有移植指征[9]。所以在低危患者强调对化疗分子学疗效的评估，初次化疗前和每次化疗后均应定量检测 MRD。

复发/难治 AML 不能达到 CR 的患者造血干细胞移植尽管疗效不佳，但毕竟为患者长期存活带来希望，目前通过改进移植方案，如加强预处理强度后输注供者淋巴细胞，或以 MRD 和 GVHD 指导下的多次 DLI 等措施明显提高了患者长期存活率[10]。针对特定患者是否实施挽救性移植要结合患者一般情况进行个体化评估。鼓励患者参加临床试验。

单倍型相合供者、非血缘供者和同胞相合移植的疗效相似[1-10]，所有适应证没有根据移植供者来源分层。

1.2 急性淋巴细胞白血病（≤65岁）

疾病分层	年龄分层	疾病状态	I级推荐	II级推荐	III级推荐
Ph+ALL	成人	CR1	Allo-HSCT（2A类）		
		≥CR2	Allo-HSCT（2A类）		
		复发/难治	减瘤后进行挽救性Allo-HSCT（2A类）		
	青少年	CR1	Allo-HSCT（2A类）		
		≥CR2	Allo-HSCT（2A类）		
		复发/难治	减瘤后进行挽救性Allo-HSCT（2A类）		
	儿童	CR1	Allo-HSCT，尤其对泼尼松反应不佳和治疗后4~12周任何时间点MRD阳性（2A类）		
		≥CR2	Allo-HSCT（2A类）		
		复发/难治	减瘤后进行挽救性Allo-HSCT（2A类）		

急性淋巴细胞白血病（≤65 岁）（续）

疾病分层	年龄分层	疾病状态	I 级推荐	II 级推荐	III 级推荐
Ph-ALL	成人	CR1	1. 成年高危 ALL 推荐 CR1 Allo-HSCT（2A 类） 2. 成年标危 ALL 推荐 CR1 Allo-HSCT（2A 类）		
		≥CR2	Allo-HSCT（2A 类）		
		复发/难治	B-ALL 减瘤后进行挽救性 Allo-HSCT（2A 类）		T-ALL 减瘤后挽救性移植（3 类）
	青少年	CR1	具备下列情况之一的青少年 ALL CR1 期移植： ● 高危 ALL 患者在 CR1 移植（2A 类） ● 标危 ALL 达到 CR 后 MRD 阳性在 CR1 移植（2A 类） ● 未采用儿童方案或加强化疗的青少年在 CR1 移植（2A 类）		
		≥CR2	Allo-HSCT（2A 类）		
		复发/难治	B-ALL 减瘤后进行挽救性 Allo-HSCT（2A 类）		T-ALL 减瘤后挽救性移植（3 类）

异基因造血干细胞移植

急性淋巴细胞白血病（≤65岁）（续）

疾病分层	年龄分层	疾病状态	Ⅰ级推荐	Ⅱ级推荐	Ⅲ级推荐
Ph-ALL	儿童	CR1	具备以下情况之一具有移植指征（2A类） ● 1个疗程诱导化疗结束时未达血液学缓解 ● 巩固化疗结束时MRD未转阴治疗中MRD转阳 ● MLL基因重排阳性		
		≥CR2	Allo-HSCT（2A类）		
		复发/难治	B-ALL减瘤后进行挽救性Allo-HSCT（2A类）		T-ALL减瘤后挽救性移植（3类）

【注释】

在酪氨酸激酶抑制剂（TKI）时代，无论成人、青少年和儿童费城染色体阳性（Ph+）的急性淋巴细胞白血病（ALL），移植仍然显示出明显的生存获益，在降低复发率、提高无病生存率上具有明显优势。[11]

成人 Ph-ALL 标危患者 CR1 期移植优于化疗，国内多个大型队列研究和病例对照研究报告均支持这个观点[12-13]。一项多中心回顾性研究对标危成人 ALL-CR1 患者移植进行预后分析，127 例为单倍体移植，144 例为同胞相合移植，77 例为非血缘移植，三组移植患者的重度 aGVHD、5 年移植相关死亡率（TRM）、5 年复发率、OS、LFS、无 GVHD 无复发存活率（GRFS）差异均无统计学意义[12]。一项多中心前瞻性Ⅲ期临床研究，年轻成人标危 ALL-CR1 患者，55 例接受了成人强化化疗方案，59 例接受了单倍体造血干细胞移植，与化疗组相比，移植组患者 2 年复发率低（12.8% vs. 46.7%）、2 年 LFS 高（80.9% vs. 51.1%）、2 年 OS 高（91.2% vs. 75.7%），差异均有统计学意义[13]。对于标危青少年采用儿童方案化疗的患者不建议在 CR1 移植。

成人 Ph-ALL 高危患者在 CR1 移植是标准治疗，移植前争取达到 MRD 阴性可以改善移植疗效，在配型相合的移植中，移植前 MRD 阴性复发率明显减低，而单倍体移植可以具有更强的 GVL 效应。

儿童 CR1 异基因移植主要用于对化疗反应不佳的患者，MRD 监测可以筛选出复发高危患者。WANG 等[14]通过对 1 126 例儿童患者的分析，发现儿童 ALL 治疗后，MRD>0.01% 作为阳性界值，可以预测患者的预后。对于儿童 Ph+ALL 患者，HSCT 同样改善了 OS 和 LFS[15]。

复发 / 难治 B-ALL 强行移植效果欠佳，如果采用新的治疗手段减瘤，甚至达到 CR 或 MRD 转阴，移植治疗疗效显著。这些新的治疗手段为抗体或细胞疗法，如 CD19-CAR-T 或 CD19/CD22CAR-T、CD19/CD3 双特异性抗体 Blinatumonmab[16-17]等，鼓励患者参加临床试验。复发 / 难治 T-ALL 强行移植预后极差，鼓励患者参加临床试验，是否移植要根据患者疾病状况和身体状况进行个性化评估。

1.3 慢性髓性白血病（≤65岁）

疾病分期	I级推荐	II级推荐	III级推荐
慢性期（CP）	慢性期具备下列情况之一有移植指征： • 对一代和二代 TKI 都耐药（2A类） • 对所有 TKI 都不耐受（2A类） • 出现 *T315i* 突变（2A类）		
加速期（AP）	加速期有移植指征，尤其是 TKI 治疗中由慢性期进展到加速期（2A类）		
急变期（BC）	急变期均具有移植指征（2A类） 急变期争取达到 CR 或 CP2 后移植（2A类）		不能达到 CR 或 CP 鼓励患者加入临床试验，包括强行移植（3类）

【注释】

靶向药物 TKI 的应用使异基因移植成为治疗慢性粒细胞白血病（CML）慢性期患者的二线选择。当患者对所有可获得的 TKIs 均耐药或不耐受，才具有在慢性期移植的指征；在发生 *T315i* 突变的慢性期患者，可以首选异基因造血干细胞移植。CML 在 TKI 治疗后的疗效反应标准见附录 2。

CML 慢性期患者移植疗效最佳，其次为加速期，最差的为急性期。所以 CML 患者服 TKI 药物期间应该定期评估效果，如病情进展到加速期应该尽早接受移植[18]，一旦进入急变期，Allo-HSCT 是唯一治愈的手段，移植前争取 CR 或达到 CP 2 期。

CML 急淋变的患者，如果 TKI 耐药，可予化疗、CAR-T 或 Blinatumonmab 治疗后进行异基因造血干细胞的移植。

1.4 骨髓增生异常综合征（≤65岁）

MDS 分层	I 级推荐	II 级推荐	III 级推荐
较高危	IPSS 中危-2 组和高危组（2A 类） IPSS-R 中危组、高危组和极高危组（2A 类） WPSS 高危和极高危组（2A 类）		
较低危	较低危组中，伴有严重血细胞减少，经其他治疗无效或伴有不良预后的遗传学异常（如 -7、3q26 重排、*TP53* 基因突变、复杂核型、单体核型）具有移植指征（2A 类）		

【注释】

MDS 的预后积分系统 IPSS、IPSS-R 和 WPSS 分别见附录 3~附录 5。

Allo-HSCT 是进展型 MDS 的常规治疗，也是唯一的治愈手段，推荐用于 IPSS 中危-2 组及高危组、IPSS-R 中危组和高危组及极高危组患者、WPSS 高危和极高危组患者。对幼稚细胞增高的 MDS 患者，移植前进行化疗或去甲基化药物是否获益存在争议，更多证据支持直接移植。刘子娴等回顾性分析 165 例同胞相合异基因移植的数据，多因素分析 HCT 合并症指数是 OS 的独立影响因素，移植前化疗和去甲基化药物对预后没有影响，作者认为 MDS-RAEB 和继发白血病没有从移植前的减瘤治疗中获益[19]。孙于谦等分析了 228 例患者的资料，得出同样结论[20]。

1.5 多发性骨髓瘤

MM	I级推荐	II级推荐	III级推荐
年轻高危			年轻，具有高危细胞遗传学[如t（4；14）；t（14；16）；17p-]（2B类）
复发/难治		复发/难治MM，尤其是自体移植后复发，具有接受异基因移植的指征（2A类）	
原发浆细胞白血病	原发浆细胞白血病可接受异基因造血干细胞移植（2A类）		

【注释】

对于适合移植的新诊断的多发性骨髓瘤患者，经有效的诱导治疗后应将自体造血干细胞移植作为首选。尽管异基因移植带来移植物抗骨髓瘤效应可能获得疾病的长久控制甚至根治，但对于新诊断

MM 在诱导治疗后采用或自体移植后序贯采用异基因造血干细胞移植是否能改善患者的远期生存仍存在争议。根据 meta 分析的结果,与串联自体移植相比,在自体移植后序贯异基因造血干细胞移植虽然能获得更好的完全缓解率,但被较高的治疗相关死亡所抵消,两组患者的无事件生存和总生存均没有统计学差异[21]。

复发/难治的多发性骨髓瘤患者,可将异基因造血干细胞移植作为挽救治疗选择之一。

1.6 淋巴瘤

1.6.1 慢性淋巴细胞白血病/小淋巴细胞淋巴瘤(CLL/SLL)

CLL	Ⅰ级推荐	Ⅱ级推荐	Ⅲ级推荐
难治			难治 CLL/SLL 患者可考虑异基因造血干细胞移植(3类)
Ritcher 转化		Ritcher 转化患者可考虑接受异基因造血干细胞移植(2A类)	

【注释】

无明显合并症,对共价结合的 BTK 抑制剂和 BCL-2 抑制剂耐药的 CLL/SLL 患者,可考虑接受异基因造血干细胞移植。

1.6.2 其他 B 细胞淋巴瘤(≤65 岁)

疾病分类	疾病状态分层	Ⅰ级推荐	Ⅱ级推荐	Ⅲ级推荐
DLBCL	≥CR2			Allo-HSCT(2B 类)
	复发/难治			含有利妥昔单抗的化学免疫治疗后≤12 个月内复发/难治患者,可以考虑接受 Allo-HSCT(2B 类)
套细胞淋巴瘤	一线治疗后 CR/PR,伴 *TP53* 突变			Allo-HSCT(2B 类)
	复发/难治			复发/难治的高危套细胞淋巴瘤,可以考虑接受 Allo-HSCT(2B 类)
伯基特淋巴瘤	≥CR2/PR			Allo-HSCT(2B 类)
	复发/难治		Allo-HSCT(2A 类)	

【注释】

1. 基于一项国际登记组的回顾性研究，对于自体移植后复发的 DLBCL 患者，403 例接受 RIC 异基因造血干细胞移植（其中 54.6% 的患者移植前处于再次完全缓解状态），1 年的复发率、非复发死亡率、无病生存率和总生存率分别为 26.2%、20%、65.6% 和 53.8%，而接受 CAR-T 治疗的患者则分别为 39.5%、4.8%、73.4% 和 55.7%。对于移植前未缓解/未治疗的患者，移植后 1 年无进展生存率和总生存率分别为 37.6% 和 49%，接受 CAR-T 治疗的患者相应结果分别为 51.5% 和 71%。这提示异基因移植可用于复发/难治 DLBCL 患者[22]。

2. 基于一项回顾性研究，42 例合并 TP53 的套细胞淋巴瘤患者（仅 1 例患者移植前处于 SD/PR 状态），接受异基因造血干细胞移植后 2 年总生存率和复发率分别为 78% 和 19%，与 TP53 阴性的患者相似[23]。

3. 基于一项系统综述，对于复发/难治的套细胞淋巴瘤患者，异基因移植后总生存率为 43%，无事件生存/无进展生存率为 34%，非复发死亡率为 30%[24]。

4. 基于一项国际登记组的回顾性研究，对于伯基特淋巴瘤患者，在 CR1、≥CR2 以及没获得 CR 时接受异基因造血干细胞移植，5 年复发率分别为 27%、49% 和 54%，5 年 OS 分别为 53%、28% 和 12%，而自体移植的患者，相应的 5 年复发率分别为 18%、50% 和 67%，5 年 OS 分别为 83%、53% 和 22%[25]。

1.6.3 T 细胞淋巴瘤（≤65 岁）

疾病分类	疾病状态分层	I 级推荐	II 级推荐	III 级推荐
侵袭性外周 T 细胞淋巴瘤（不包括 ALK+ 间变大细胞淋巴瘤）	获得治疗反应		高危 T 细胞淋巴瘤患者，在获得治疗反应后接受 Allo-HSCT 治疗（2A 类）	
	复发/难治		Allo-HSCT（2A 类）	
ALK+ 间变大细胞淋巴瘤	复发/难治			Allo-HSCT（3 类）
NK/T 细胞淋巴瘤	获得治疗反应			晚期，或者 PINK 评分高危患者，可以接受 Allo-HSCT（2B 类）
	复发/难治		Allo-HSCT（2A 类）	

【注释】

1. 基于一项国际多中心 III 期临床研究，对于有高危因素的外周 T 细胞淋巴瘤（不包含 ALK+ 间变大细胞淋巴瘤），在疾病控制及以上（CR/CRu/PR/SD）的患者，随机接受自体移植和异基因造血干细胞移植，中位随访 42 个月，异基因移植和自体移植组 3 年无事件生存分别为 43% 和 38%，3 年无进展生存分别为 43% 和 39%。对于达到 PR 以上的患者，异基因移植后无一例复发，而自体移植后 1 年累积复发率为 36%，异基因移植组和自体移植组移植后 1 年非复发死亡率分别为 23% 和 0[26]。

2. 对于复发/难治外周 T 细胞淋巴瘤，异基因移植后 3 年非复发死亡率、总生存率、无进展生存率分别为 32%、50% 和 42%，自体移植后 3 年非复发死亡率、总生存率、无进展生存率分别为 7%、55% 和 41%，但对于移植前未获得 CR 的患者，异基因移植的 3 年 OS 优于自体移植[27]。

1.7 重型再生障碍性贫血（≤60岁）

年龄分层	疾病分层	Ⅰ级推荐	Ⅱ级推荐	Ⅲ级推荐
≤50岁	新诊断 SAA/vSAA	1. 造血干细胞移植为一线治疗选择（2A类） 2. allo-HSCT 时首选 HLA 完全相合的同胞供者（2A类）；如果没有完全相合的同胞供者，单倍体相合移植和 10/10 相合非血缘移植均可（2A类）		非血缘脐带血移植（3类）
	IST 治疗失败的 SAA/vSAA 或从非 SAA 进展的 SAA/vSAA	1. 造血干细胞移植为首选（2A类） 2. allo-HSCT 时首选 HLA 全合的同胞供者（2A类） 3. 如果没有完全相合的同胞供者，单倍体供者移植和 10/10 相合非血缘供者移植均为可选（2A类）		非血缘脐带血移植（3类）
50~60岁	新诊断 SAA/vSAA	1. allo-HSCT 为二线治疗选择（2A类） 2. allo-HSCT 时首选同胞相合供者（2A类） 如果没有完全相合的同胞供者，单倍体相合移植和 10/10 相合非血缘供者均为可选（2A类）		非血缘脐血供者（3类）
	IST 治疗失败的 SAA/vSAA 或由非 SAA 进展的 SAA/vSAA	1. allo-HSCT 为首选治疗（2A类） 2. allo-HSCT 时首选同胞相合供者（2A类） 如果没有完全相合的同胞供者，单倍体相合供者和 10/10 相合非血缘供者均为可选（2A类）		非血缘脐血供者（3类）

注：SAA/vSAA. 重症再生障碍性贫血/极重症再生障碍性贫血；allo-HSCT. 异基因造血干细胞移植；IST. 免疫抑制剂治疗。

【注释】

黄晓军等建立了基于 G-CSF/ATG 的非体外去 T 单倍体造血干细胞移植治疗 SAA/vSAA 的模式,并组织实施了全国多中心研究验证了该方案的疗效,长期随访研究显示 haplo-HSCT 用于免疫抑制剂治疗失败的 SAA/vSAA,在儿童和成人患者中 9 年 OS 分别达 90.1% 和 80.8%,9 年 FFS 分别达 88.7% 和 79.4%[28];用于一线治疗 SAA/vSAA,haplo-HSCT 取得了和同胞相合移植相似的疗效。

3 年 OS 率分别为 86.1% 和 91.3%,3 年 FFS 率分别为 85.0% 和 89.8%[29]。刘立民等报道一线治疗 haplo-HSCT 与一线免疫抑制剂治疗(IST)用于 SAA/vSAA,无失败存活率(FFS)和生活质量 haplo-HSCT 都明显优于 IST 组[30]。刘立民等报道从 non-SAA 进展而来的 SAA/vSAA,allo-HSCT 疗效明显优于 IST,而且配型相合同胞、全相合非血缘和单倍体移植疗效类似,所以从 non-SAA 发展来的 SAA/vSAA 患者应首先考虑移植[31]。

本指南以 50 岁年龄为界,≤50 岁 SAA 患者首选 allo-HSCT,haplo-HSCT、10/10 相合的非血缘移植与同胞相合移植疗效相似,由此,当患者没有配型相合同胞供者时,haplo-HSCT 可作为一线治疗应用。年龄超过 50 岁的患者,一般将 allo-HSCT 作为二线选择,即 IST 治疗失败后再进行移植。关于移植时机的探讨,许兰平等报道在 haplo-HSCT 治疗 SAA 时预测移植相关死亡率(TRM)的模型并在独立的患者群进行了验证,发现影响 TRM 的因素有三个,分别为移植前病程长于 12 个月、ECOG 大于 2 和造血干细胞移植合并症指数(HCT-CI)大于 1[32],所以采用 IST 治疗的患者,要适时评估疗效,不要错过最佳移植时机。

参考文献

[1] HUANG XJ, ZHU HH, CHANG YJ, et al. The superiority of haploidentical related stem cell transplantation over chemotherapy alone as post remission treatment for patients with intermediate-or high-risk acute myeloid leukemia in first complete remission. Blood, 2012, 119 (23): 5584-5590.

[2] YU S, HUANG F, WANG Y, et al. Haploidentical transplantation might have superior graft-versus-leukemia effect than HLA-matched sibling transplantation for high-risk acute myeloid leukemia in first complete remission: A prospective multicentre cohort study. Leukemia, 2020, 34 (5): 1433-1443.

[3] WANG Y, LIU QF, XU LP, et al. Haploidentical vs identical-sibling transplant for AML in remission: A multicenter, prospective study. Blood, 2015, 125 (25): 3956-3962.

[4] LV M, WANG Y, CHANG YJ, et al. Myeloablative haploidentical transplantation is superior to chemotherapy for patients with intermediate-risk acute myelogenous leukemia in first complete remission. Clin Cancer Res, 2019, 25 (6): 1737-1748.

[5] ZHU HH, ZHANG XH, QIN YZ, et al. MRD-directed risk stratification treatment may improve outcomes of t (8; 21) AML in the first complete remission: Results from the AML05 multicenter trial. Blood, 2013, 121 (20): 4056-4062.

[6] HU GH, CHENG YF, LU AD, et al. Allogeneic hematopoietic stem cell transplantation can improve the prognosis of high-risk pediatric t (8; 21) acute myeloid leukemia in first remission based on MRD-guided treatment. BMC Cancer, 2020, 20 (1): 553.

[7] DUAN W, LIU X, JIA J, et al. The loss or absence of minimal residual disease of <0.1% at any time after two cycles

of consolidation chemotherapy in CBFB-MYH11-positive acute myeloid leukaemia indicates poor prognosis. Br J Haematol, 2021, 192 (2): 265-271.

[8] DENG DX, ZHU HH, LIU YR, et al. Minimal residual disease detected by multiparameter flow cytometry is complementary to genetics for risk stratification treatment in acute myeloid leukemia with biallelic CEBPA mutations. Leuk Lymphoma, 2019, 60 (9): 2181-2189.

[9] 赵婷, 主鸿鹄, 王婧, 等. 早期评估NPM1突变阳性急性髓系白血病患者残留白血病水平的预后意义. 中华血液学杂志, 2017, 38 (1): 10-16.

[10] YU S, HUANG F, FAN Z, et al. Haploidentical versus HLA-matched sibling transplantation for refractory acute leukemia undergoing sequential intensified conditioning followed by DLI: An analysis from two prospective data. J Hematol Oncol, 2020, 13 (1): 18.

[11] XUE YJ, CHENG YF, LU AD, et al. Allogeneic hematopoietic stem cell transplantation, especially haploidentical, may improve long-term survival for high-risk pediatric patients with Philadelphia chromosome-positive acute lymphoblastic leukemia in the tyrosine kinase inhibitor era. Biol Blood Marrow Transplant, 2019, 25 (8): 1611-1620.

[12] HAN LJ, WANG Y, FAN ZP, et al. Haploidentical transplantation compared with matched sibling and unrelated donor transplantation for adults with standard-risk acute lymphoblastic leukaemia in first complete remission. Br J Haematol, 2017, 179 (1): 120-130.

[13] LV M, JIANG Q, ZHOU DB, et al. Comparison of haplo-SCT and chemotherapy for young adults with standard-risk Ph-negative acute lymphoblastic leukemia in CR1. J Hematol Oncol, 2020, 13 (1): 52.

[14] WANG Y, XUE YJ, JIA YP, et al. Re-emergence of minimal residual disease detected by flow cytometry predicts an adverse outcome in pediatric acute lymphoblastic leukemia. Front Oncol, 2020, 10: 596677.

[15] XUE YJ, SUO P, HUANG XJ, et al. Superior survival of unmanipulated haploidentical haematopoietic stem cell transplantation compared with intensive chemotherapy as post-remission treatment for children with very high-risk

philadelphia chromosome negative B-cell acute lymphoblastic leukaemia in first complete remission. Br J Haematol, 2020, 188 (5): 757-767.

[16] ZHAO H, WEI J, WEI G, et al. Pre-transplant MRD negativity predicts favorable outcomes of CAR-T therapy followed by haploidentical HSCT for relapsed/refractory acute lymphoblastic leukemia: A multi-center retrospective study. J Hematol Oncol, 2020, 13 (1): 42.

[17] WANG N, HU X, CAO W, et al. Efficacy and safety of CAR19/22 T-cell cocktail therapy in patients with refractory/relapsed B-cell malignancies. Blood, 2020, 135 (1): 17-27.

[18] XU L, ZHU H, HU J, et al. Superiority of allogeneic hematopoietic stem cell transplantation to nilotinib and dasatinib for adult patients with chronic myelogenous leukemia in the accelerated phase. Front Med, 2015, 9 (3): 304-311.

[19] 刘子娴, 吕梦楠, 王茜茜, 等. 异基因造血干细胞移植治疗骨髓增生异常综合征的预后因素分析. 中华血液学杂志, 2019, 40 (6): 484-489.

[20] SUN YQ, XU LP, LIU KY, et al. Pre-transplantation cytoreduction does not benefit advanced myelodysplastic syndrome patients after myeloablative transplantation with grafts from family donors. Cancer Commun (Lond), 2021, 41 (4): 333-344.

[21] KHARFAN-DABAJA MA, HAMADANI M, RELJIC T, et al. Comparative efficacy of tandem autologous versus autologous followed by allogeneic hematopoietic cell transplantation in patients with newly diagnosed multiple myeloma: A systematic review and meta-analysis of randomized controlled trials. J Hematol Oncol, 2013, 6: 2.

[22] HAMADANI M, GOPAL AK, PASQUINI M, et al. Allogeneic transplant and CAR-T therapy after autologous transplant failure in DLBCL: A noncomparative cohort analysis. Blood Adv, 2022, 6 (2): 486-494.

[23] LIN RJ, HO C, HILDEN PD, et al. Allogeneic haematopoietic cell transplantation impacts on outcomes of mantle cell lymphoma with TP53 alterations. Br J Haematol, 2019, 184 (6): 1006-1010.

[24] KHARFAN-DABAJA MA, RELJIC T, EL-ASMAR J, et al. Reduced-intensity or myeloablative allogeneic hemato-

poietic cell transplantation for mantle cell lymphoma: A systematic review. Future Oncol, 2016, 12 (22): 2631-2642.

[25] MARAMATTOM LV, HARI PN, BURNS LJ, et al. Autologous and allogeneic transplantation for burkitt lymphoma outcomes and changes in utilization: A report from the center for international blood and marrow transplant research. Biol Blood Marrow Transplant, 2013, 19 (2): 173-179.

[26] SCHMITZ N, TRUEMPER L, BOUABDALLAH K, et al. A randomized phase 3 trial of autologous vs allogeneic transplantation as part of first-line therapy in poor-risk peripheral T-NHL. Blood, 2021, 137 (19): 2646-2656.

[27] DU J, YU D, HAN X, et al. Comparison of allogeneic stem cell transplant and autologous stem cell transplant in refractory or relapsed peripheral T-cell lymphoma: A systematic review and meta-analysis. JAMA Netw Open, 2021, 4 (5): e219807.

[28] XU LP, XU ZL, WANG SQ, et al. Long-term follow-up of haploidentical transplantation in relapsed/refractory severe aplastic anemia: A multicenter prospective study. Science Bulletin, 2022 [2023-03-01] https://doi.org/10.1016/j.scib.2022.01.024.

[29] XU LP, JIN S, WANG SQ, et al. Upfront haploidentical transplant for acquired severe aplastic anemia: Registry-based comparison with matched related transplant. J Hematol Oncol, 2017, 10 (1): 25.

[30] LIU L, ZHANG Y, JIAO W, et al. Comparison of efficacy and health-related quality of life of first-line haploidentical hematopoietic stem cell transplantation with unrelated cord blood infusion and first-line immunosuppressive therapy for acquired severe aplastic anemia. Leukemia, 2020, 34 (12): 3359-3369.

[31] LIU L, ZHAO X, MIAO M, et al. Inefficacy of immunosuppressive therapy for severe aplastic anemia progressing from Non-SAA: Improved outcome after allogeneic hematopoietic stem cell transplantation. Front Oncol, 2021, 11: 739561.

[32] XU LP, YU Y, CHENG YF, et al. Development and validation of a mortality predicting scoring system for severe aplastic anaemia patients receiving haploidentical allogeneic transplantation. Br J Haematol, 2022, 196 (3): 735-742.

2 异基因造血干细胞移植治疗血液系统疾病的供者选择

2.1 供者来源选择

	Ⅰ级推荐	Ⅱ级推荐	Ⅲ级推荐
HLA全相合同胞供者	大多数情况下为首选供者（2A类）		
单倍型相合供者	无HLA全相合同胞供者时作为首选供者，尤其对于有复发高风险需要紧急移植的患者（2A类）	有HLA全相合同胞供者时，在单倍型相合移植经验丰富的移植单位：急性白血病移植前微小残留病阳性等高复发风险患者，可优选单倍型相合供者；对于年龄>50岁急性白血病患者，可优选子女供者（1B类）	
非血缘自愿供者	无HLA全相合同胞供者且不是复发高风险需要紧急移植的患者，根据患者意愿，作为可选供者（2A类）		
非血缘脐带血供者	无HLA全相合同胞供者的儿童患者，据患者意愿作为可选供者（2A类）		

【注释】

目前,供者来源呈现多样化,移植患者可能面临多个备选供者。在没有 HLA 全相合的同胞供者时,替代供者的选择应结合患者情况(是否有复发高危风险、年龄、身体状况)、移植单位的经验及供者特异性 HLA 抗体综合考虑,还应考虑:①各供者来源的优缺点,影响预后的因素因供者来源不同而异;②各中心的优势和特色[1-4]。

在有 HLA 全相合的同胞供者时,优选单倍型相合供者的情况基于生物随机研究[5-8],且得到基本一致的专家共识度[9-10],尤其对于开展单倍型相合移植经验丰富的移植单位,故本指南将其作为ⅠB级推荐。在基于供受者年龄、性别、血型相合为核心的供者选择积分体系中,危险积分高的 HLA 全合同胞供者移植疗效差于危险积分低的单倍型相合供者[11]。

在没有 HLA 全相合的同胞供者,且无同胞、子女、父母年迈体弱或过世或单倍型相合供者的供者特异性抗 HLA 抗体(DSA)强阳性时,非血缘志愿供者作为备选供者;反之亦然[12]。但目前尚无强有力的循证医学证据,故本指南将其作为Ⅲ级推荐。

2.2 非体外去除T细胞单倍型相合供者选择

	I级推荐	II级推荐	III级推荐
供者特异性抗HLA抗体（DSA）	尽量避免DSA阳性供者（2A类）	DSA平均荧光强度（MFI）≥10 000的患者尽量更换供者对于无供者可更换的患者，对DSA进行处理可选血浆置换、静脉人血免疫球蛋白、CD20单克隆抗体和硼替佐米等方法（2A类）	
供者年龄	年轻优于年长供者（2A类）		
供者性别	男性优于女性供者（2A类）	男性患者，男性供者优于女性供者（2A类）	
供受者亲属关系	子女或年轻同胞优于父母供者；"北京方案"中父亲优于母亲；一级亲属优于二级亲属（2A类）	男性患者，父亲优于年长的女性同胞供者（2A类）	

非体外去除 T 细胞单倍型相合供者选择（续）

	I 级推荐	II 级推荐	III 级推荐
ABO 血型	ABO 血型相合优于次要不合，次要不合优于主要不合（2A 类）		
非遗传性母亲抗原（NIMA）	非遗传性母亲抗原（NIMA）不合的同胞优于非遗传性父亲抗原（NIPA）不合的同胞（2A 类）		
巨细胞病毒（CMV）血清抗体	供受者 CMV IgG 抗体阳性供阳性，阴性供阴性（2A 类）	后置环磷酰胺方案，受者 CMV IgG 抗体阳性，供者阳性、阴性均可（2A 类）	"北京方案"中受者 CMV IgG 抗体阳性，尽量选择阳性供者（2B 类）

【注释】

目前，不同中心判定 DSA 阳性的 MFI 阈值不同。常英军等发现 DSA MFI ≥ 2 000 与植入不良密切相关，MFI ≥ 10 000 与移植排斥密切相关。对于 DSA 阳性的患者而言，可以考虑更换供者。对于无供者可更换的患者，可以考虑应用血浆置换、静脉人血免疫球蛋白、CD20 单克隆抗体和硼替佐米等方法[13-15]。但目前尚无DSA阳性最佳处理方法的高级别循证医学证据，故本指南对于DSA阳性的处理作为Ⅱ级推荐。

由于供受者年龄、性别与供受者亲属关系间的紧密关联导致的比较分析的复杂性，结果来源于大型回顾性研究的亚组分析[16]，且在不同的疾病中结果不尽相同[17]，故本指南对于供受者性别和亲属关系的亚组作为Ⅱ级推荐。一级亲属优于二级亲属[18]、NIMA[19]供者的选择虽然仅来源于大型回顾性研究，但"北京方案"专家共识度高[20]，而杀伤免疫球蛋白受体（KIR）[21]对移植疗效的影响结果不一。

后置环磷酰胺（PTCY）模式下受者CMV血清学阳性时供者的选择仅来源于回顾性研究，且专家共识度稍低，故本指南将其作为Ⅱ级推荐。因我国人群CMV血清学阳性率在90%以上，"北京方案"下受者CMV血清学阳性时供者的选择仅来源于病例-对照研究，故本指南将其作为Ⅲ级推荐。

总之，非体外去T单倍型相合移植疗效不再依赖于HLA不合的程度，供者选择应考虑年龄、性别、ABO、DSA、NIMA、KIR、CMV等（附：单倍型相合供者选择原则）。另外，还需要考虑：①影响预后的供者因素因单倍型移植模式不同而异，应考虑患者所处的移植模式；②随着移植技术的不断改进，某些供者特征可能会失去对移植预后影响的价值，而新的供者特征会被发现，因此供者选择原则会不断更新。

附：单倍型相合供者选择原则

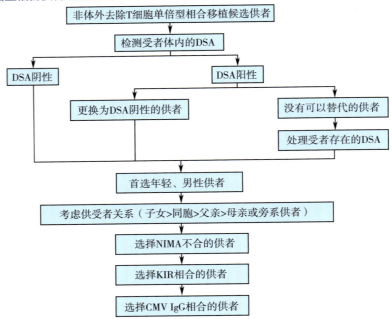

2.3 非血缘志愿者供者选择

	Ⅰ级推荐	Ⅱ级推荐	Ⅲ级推荐
HLA 配型	优选 HLA-A、-B、-C 和 -DRB1 高分辨 8/8 相合供者；次选高分辨 7/8 相合供者（2A 类）	当在几个 8/8（10/10）或 7/8（9/10）供者中选择时，考虑 HLA-DPB1 相合（12/12）或可允许错配（尤其是 TCE3 核心等位基因）的供者；尽量减少 HLA-DRB3/4/5 和 HLA-DQB1 的不匹配（2A 类）	
DSA	尽量避免 DSA 阳性供者（2A 类）	DSA 阳性患者尽量更换供者（2A 类）	
供者年龄	年轻供者优于年长供者（2A 类）		
供者性别		男性供者优于女性供者（2A 类）	
ABO 血型		ABO 血型相合优于次要不合，次要不合优于主要不合（2A 类）	
CMV 血清抗体		供受者 CMV IgG 抗体阴性供阴性，阳性供阳性（2A 类）	

【注释】

非血缘志愿者供者（URD）移植中，供受者间 HLA-A、-B、-C、-DRB1 配型是首要考虑因素。当有若干个 8/8HLA 相合的 URD 可供选择时，供者年龄是影响预后的最重要因素。在恶性疾病中，功能匹配通过识别可容许的、低风险的 HLA-DPB1 差异可以改善预后[22]（附：非血缘志愿者供者选择原则）。本指南以国家骨髓捐献者计划（NMDP）的指南中 URD 的选择为参考[23]，但在新的免疫抑制剂时代，组织相容性的作用可能会发生重大改变，因此不应视其为一成不变的。

除供者年龄之外的其他非 HLA 供者因素，多来源于回顾性研究，且由于不同研究的结论不一致，美国国家骨髓库的指南未给出具体建议，故本指南将其作为 II 级推荐。KIR 在 URD 移植中的作用仍存在争议。

附：非血缘志愿者供者选择原则

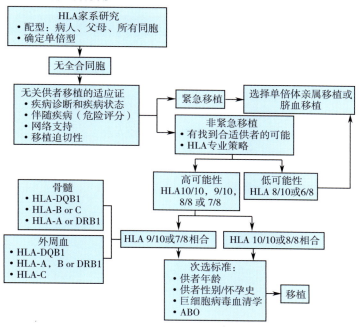

2.4 非血缘脐带血供者选择

	I 级推荐	II 级推荐	III 级推荐
HLA 配型	优选 HLA-A、-B、-C 和 -DRB1 高分辨 8/8 相合供者；次选高分辨 7/8 相合供者；三选高分辨 6/8 或 5/8 相合供者（2A 类）		
冷冻保存细胞数量	1. 单份 UCBT*：TNC 恶性病 ≥（2.5~3）× 10^7/kg，SAA ≥ 5 × 10^7/kg 和/或 CD34+ 细胞 ≥ 1.5 × 10^5/kg； 2. 双份 UCBT：每份 TNC ≥ 1.5 × 10^7/kg 和/或 CD34+ 细胞 ≥ 1 × 10^5/kg；双份之和 TNC ≥ 3.5 × 10^7/kg 和/或 CD34+ 细胞 ≥ 1.8 × 10^5/kg		
脐带血库认证			优先选择受认证的脐带血库（2B 类）

非血缘脐带血供者选择(续)

	I 级推荐	II 级推荐	III 级推荐
DSA		优先考虑HLA配型和细胞数量的前提下尽量避免DSA阳性供者(2A类)	
ABO血型		ABO血型相合优于次要不合,次要不合优于主要不合(2A类)	

注:TNC.总有核细胞数(total number of nucleated cells);UCB.脐带血(umbilical cord blood);UCBT.脐带血移植(umbilical cord blood transplantation)。* 如果在单份UCBT未能达到所需最小细胞数,需考虑双份UCBT。

【注释】

非血缘脐带血（UCB）供者移植中，供受者间 HLA-A、-B、-C、-DRB1 配型和冻存细胞剂量是首要考虑因素，且与移植适应证即疾病类型、患者体重相关。本指南以欧洲脐血移植协作组（Eurocord）脐带血选择标准[24]（附：非血缘脐带血供者选择原则）和国家骨髓捐献者计划（NMDP）指南中 UCB 的选择为参考[23]。NMDP 建议：儿童或小体重成人，TNC ≥（2.5~3）× 10^7/kg，CD34 ≥ $2 × 10^5$/kg 时优先选择 HLA 相合度高的；成人和大体重儿童选择脐血时细胞数优先于 HLA 相合度[23]。

ABO 血型相合程度多来源于回顾性研究，且由于不同研究的结论不一致，故本指南将其作为 Ⅱ 级推荐。目前没有足够的数据支持 NIMA 或 KIR 的情况进行选择。

附：非血缘脐带血供者选择原则

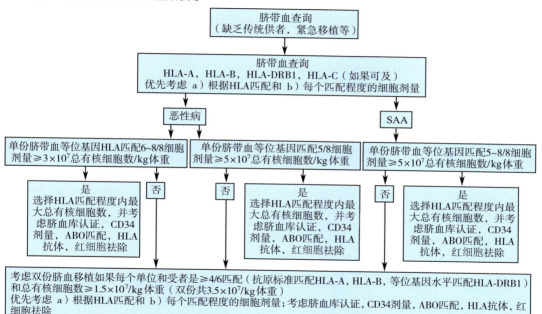

参考文献

[1] LV M, GORIN NC, HUANG XJ. A vision for the future of allogeneic hematopoietic stem cell transplantation in the next decade. Sci Bull (Beijing), 2022, 67 (19): 1921-1924.

[2] MO XD, TANG BL, ZHANG XH, et al. Comparison of outcomes after umbilical cord blood and unmanipulated haploidentical hematopoietic stem cell transplantation in children with high-risk acute lymphoblastic leukemia. Int J Cancer, 2016, 139 (9): 2106-2115.

[3] XU LP, XU ZL, WANG SQ, et al. Long-term follow-up of haploidentical transplantation in relapsed/refractory severe aplastic anemia: A multicenter prospective study, Science Bulletin, 2022 [2023-03-01] https://doi.org/10.1016/j.scib.2022.01.024.

[4] GAO L, ZHANG C, GAO L, et al. Favorable outcome of haploidentical hematopoietic stem cell, transplantation in Philadelphia chromosome-positive acute lymphoblastic leukemia: A multicenter study in Southwest China. J Hematol Oncol, 2015, 8: 90.

[5] CHANG YJ, WANG Y, LIU YR, et al. Haploidentical allograft is superior to matched sibling donor allograft in eradicating pre-transplantation minimal residual disease of AML patients as determined by multiparameter flow cytometry: A retrospective and prospective analysis. J Hematol Oncol, 2017, 10 (1): 134.

[6] CHANG YJ, WANG Y, XU LP, et al. Haploidentical donor is preferred over matched sibling donor for pre-transplantation MRD positive ALL: A phase 3 genetically randomized study. J Hematol Oncol, 2020, 13 (1): 27.

[7] GUO H, CHANG YJ, HONG Y, et al. Dynamic immune profiling identifies the stronger graft-versus-leukemia (GVL) effects with haploidentical allografts compared to HLA-matched stem cell transplantation. Cell Mol

Immunol, 2021, 18 (5): 1172-1185.
[8] WANG Y, LIU QF, WU DP, et al. Improved survival after offspring donor transplant compared with older aged-matched siblings for older leukaemia patients. Br J Haematol, 2020, 189 (1): 153-161.
[9] ZHANG XH, CHEN J, HAN MZ, et al. The consensus from The Chinese Society of Hematology on indications, conditioning regimens and donor selection for allogeneic hematopoietic stem cell transplantation: 2021 update. J Hematol Oncol, 2021, 14 (1): 145.
[10] WANG Y, CHEN H, CHEN J, et al. The consensus on the monitoring, treatment, and prevention of leukemia relapse after allogeneic hematopoietic stem cell transplantation in China. Cancer Lett, 2018, 438: 63-75.
[11] WANG Y, WU DP, LIU QF, et al. Donor and recipient age, gender and ABO incompatibility regardless of donor source: Validated criteria for donor selection for haematopoietic transplants. Leukemia, 2018, 32 (2): 492-498.
[12] 常英军. 我如何选择异基因造血干细胞移植供者. 中华血液学杂志, 2016, 37 (8): 643-649.
[13] CIUREA SO, CAO K, FERNANDEZ-VINA M, et al. The European Society for Blood and Marrow Transplantation (EBMT) consensus guidelines for the detection and treatment of donor-specific anti-HLA antibodies (DSA) in haploidentical hematopoietic cell transplantation. Bone Marrow Transplant, 2018, 53 (5): 521-534.
[14] XU L, CHEN H, CHEN J, et al. The consensus on indications, conditioning regimen, and donor selection of allogeneic hematopoietic cell transplantation for hematological diseases in China-recommendations from the Chinese Society of Hematology. J Hematol Oncol, 2018, 11 (1): 33.
[15] CHANG YJ, XU LP, WANG Y, et al. Rituximab for desensitization during HLA-mismatched stem cell transplantation in patients with a positive donor-specific anti-HLA antibody. Bone Marrow Transplant, 2020, 55 (7): 1326-1336.
[16] WANG Y, CHANG YJ, XU LP, et al. Who is the best donor for a related HLA haplotype-mismatched transplant？. Blood, 2014, 124 (6): 843-850.
[17] XU LP, WANG SQ, MA YR, et al. Who is the best haploidentical donor for acquired severe aplastic anemia？:

Experience from a multicenter study. J Hematol Oncol, 2019, 12 (1): 87.
[18] MO XD, ZHANG YY, ZHANG XH, et al. The role of collateral related donors in haploidentical hematopoietic stem cell transplantation. Science Bulletin, 2018, 63 (20): 1376-1382.
[19] WANG Y, ZHAO XY, XU LP, et al. Lower incidence of acute GVHD is associated with the rapid recovery of CD4 (+) CD25 (+) CD45RA (+) regulatory T cells in patients who received haploidentical allografts from NIMA-mismatched donors: A retrospective (development) and prospective (validation) cohort-based study. Oncoimmunology, 2016, 5 (12): e1242546.
[20] CIUREA SO, AL MALKI MM, KONGTIM P, et al. The European Society for Blood and Marrow Transplantation (EBMT) consensus recommendations for donor selection in haploidentical hematopoietic cell transplantation. Bone Marrow Transplant, 2020, 55 (1): 12-24.
[21] ZHAO XY, CHANG YJ, ZHAO XS, et al. Recipient expression of ligands for donor inhibitory KIRs enhances NK-cell function to control leukemic relapse after haploidentical transplantation. Eur J Immunol, 2015, 45 (8): 2396-2408.
[22] ARRIETA-BOLAÑOS E, CRIVELLO P, HE M, et al. A core group of structurally similar HLA-DPB1 alleles drives permissiveness after hematopoietic cell transplantation. Blood, 2022, 140 (6): 659-663.
[23] DEHN J, SPELLMAN S, HURLEY CK, et al. Selection of unrelated donors and cord blood units for hematopoietic cell transplantation: Guidelines from the NMDP/CIBMTR. Blood, 2019, 134 (12): 924-934.
[24] VEYS P, DANBY R, VORA A, et al. UK experience of unrelated cord blood transplantation in paediatric patients. Br J Haematol, 2016, 172 (3): 482-486.

3 异基因造血干细胞移植前患者及供者评估

3.1 患者评估

	Ⅰ级推荐	Ⅱ级推荐	Ⅲ级推荐
病史采集及体格检查	• 完整的病史采集（病史、初治时诊断分层、既往治疗方案、疗效及疾病状态、过敏史、输血史等） • 体格检查 • 体能状态评分		
实验室检查	• HLA 分型 • 抗群体抗体和 DSA 筛查（HLA 单倍型相合及脐血移植供者需进行） • 血尿便常规 • ABO 及 Rh 血型、血型抗体效价（供受者 ABO 血型不合者） • 生化全项、凝血功能、红细胞沉降率、C 反应蛋白感染筛查（抗 HAV，乙肝五项检查，HBV-DNA，抗 HCV、HCV-RNA，艾滋病病毒，梅毒，抗 CMV-IgM、IgG，抗 EBV-IgM、IgG） • 血清铁蛋白（AA 患者） • 育龄妇女须进行妊娠试验	血气分析（移植前存在肺部疾病者）	

患者评估(续)

	I 级推荐	II 级推荐	III 级推荐
影像学检查	<ul><li>胸部 CT、腹部超声</li><li>心电图、心脏超声检查</li><li>头颅 CT 或 MRI</li><li>淋巴瘤:PET-CT</li></ul>	肺功能(儿童患者不需进行)	
专科检查	口腔科、耳鼻喉科、眼科、肛肠外科、妇科(女性患者)	心理评估(必要时) 生育咨询(必要时)	
本病评估	<ul><li>白血病和 MDS:骨髓检查包括形态、MRD 检测</li><li>AA:骨髓形态、活检、免疫分型、染色体和 MDS 相关基因,PNH 克隆检测</li><li>MM:乳酸脱氢酶、血清钙、β_2 微球蛋白、血清免疫球蛋白定量、血清蛋白电泳及血免疫固定电泳、NT-Pro-BNP 及 cTNI/TNI、24 小时尿总蛋白及白蛋白定量、24 小时尿轻链定量、尿免疫固定电泳、骨髓细胞形态学及 MRD 检测</li></ul>	染色体脆性和彗星试验(儿童或年轻 AA 患者),基因突变筛查(必要时)	
中枢神经系统白血病(CNSL)筛查	CNSL 筛查(急性白血病患者)		
造血干细胞移植合并症指数(HCT-CI)		所有受者移植前进行评估	

【注释】

移植前患者评估取决于基础疾病,在预处理前完成,评估结果可能影响移植预处理方案选择、移植供者选择和移植时机选择[1]。仔细询问和复习病史,详细了解初诊情况及对化疗的效果、初始诊断、预后分层及疗效预测,决定是否选择移植。

了解移植前疾病所处现状及 MRD 状态,完善骨髓检查(形态学、染色体分析、免疫分型、特异融合基因标志、*WT1* 基因等),AL 患者需了解 CNSL 预防及治疗情况,ALL 预防鞘内注射 4~6 次,AML 2~4 次。如确诊 CNSL 者,需要达到 CR,CML 急变患者移植前应进行 CNSL 筛查,MDS、CML-CP/AP 移植前无需进行。

淋巴瘤患者了解病理结果及疾病分期,染色体或融合基因异常情况,既往治疗及效果,是否接受放射治疗及免疫治疗,如果有放疗史,应了解放疗的累积剂量、照射野及照射时间。

AA 患者移植前需行骨髓形态、活检、免疫分型、染色体和 MDS 相关基因检查,以再次确定诊断,了解有无 PNH 克隆,既往治疗及疗效,尤其是否应用 ATG 治疗,输血史,输注血是否是辐照血。检查血清铁蛋白,了解有无血色病。对于儿童或年轻患者,应注意除外先天性贫血如范可尼贫血等,了解生长发育和智力状况,有无畸形和咖啡牛奶斑,检查染色体脆性和彗星试验,必要时进行基因突变筛查。

了解患者既往所患疾病,器官功能、既往感染或潜在感染情况评估患者耐受情况及 TRM,移植前常用造血干细胞并发症指数(HCI-CI)预测移植相关死亡率(TRM)[2-3]。移植前患者应符合条件见附录 6,HCT-CI 见附录 7。

3.2 供者移植前评估

	I 级推荐	II 级推荐	III 级推荐
实验室检查	<ul><li>HLA 分型</li><li>血尿便常规</li><li>ABO 及 Rh 血型、血型抗体效价(供受者 ABO 血型不合者)</li><li>生化全项、凝血功能</li><li>感染筛查(抗 HAV,乙肝五项检查、HBV-DNA、抗 HCV、HCV-RNA,HIV、梅毒、抗 CMV-IgM、IgG,抗 EBV-IgM、IgG)</li><li>育龄妇女须进行妊娠试验</li></ul>		
影像学检查	<ul><li>胸部 X 线或 CT</li><li>腹部超声</li><li>心电图</li></ul>		

【注释】

供者在捐献造血干细胞前 3 个月内,要全面评估身体情况,除外血液系统疾病,是否可以耐受麻醉、骨髓采集和粒细胞集落刺激因子(G-CSF)动员,是否有心脏、肝脏、肺脏和肾脏方面的疾病。HIV 感染者、严重的心脏疾病,尤其冠心病、心功能不全及严重的呼吸系统疾病、严重的脑血管疾病,如脑梗塞、脑出血病史者、血栓病、肾脏功能受损、肿瘤或肿瘤病史、活动性自身免疫性疾病、活动性结核或肝炎、妊娠期女性、精神疾病没有控制、没有行为能力者等的供者均为捐献造血干细胞的禁忌。患有结核病供者在控制结核后可以捐献。乙型肝炎患者 HBV-DNA 转阴后可以捐献。

参考文献

[1] APPELLLBAUM F R, FORMAN SJ, NEGRIN RS, et al. Thomas' Hematopoietic cell transplantation. 4th ed. Oxford: Blackwell Publishing Ltd, 2009.
[2] SORROR ML, MARIS MB, STORB R, et al. Hematopoietic cell transplantation (HCT)-specific comorbidity index: A new tool for risk assessment before allogeneic HCT. Blood, 2005, 106 (8): 2912-2919.
[3] MO XD, XU LP, LIU DH, et al. The hematopoietic cell transplantation-specific comorbidity index (HCT-CI) is an outcome predictor for partially matched related donor transplantation. Am J Hematol, 2013, 88 (6): 497-502.

4 异基因造血干细胞移植预处理方案

4.1 标准清髓性（MAC）预处理

	Ⅰ级推荐	Ⅱ级推荐	Ⅲ级推荐
AML/MDS/CML	含全身放疗预处理：Cy/TBI（1A 类）		
	化疗预处理： 　Bu/Cy（1A 类） 　Flu/Bu（2A 类） 　改良 Bu/Cy（2A 类）		
ALL	含全身放疗预处理： 　Cy/TBI（2A 类） 　Vp/TBI（2A 类）		
	化疗预处理： 　Bu/Cy（1B 类） 　改良 Bu/Cy（2A 类）		
AA	Cy+ATG（2A 类）		Flu-Cy-TBI（2B 类）

注：Bu. 白消安（busulfan）；Cy. 环磷酰胺（cyclophosphamide）；Flu. 福达拉滨（fludarabine）；TBI. 全身放疗（total body radiation）；Vp. 依托泊苷（etoposide，Vp-16）。

【注释】

清髓性预处理强度（myeloablative conditioning，MAC）具有不可逆清除宿主骨髓造血功能作用，优势为抗白血病作用强，降低移植后疾病复发率[1]。在疾病风险指数（disease risk index，DRI）低中危 AML 中，MAC 预处理显著降低 AML 移植后复发率，提高无病生存率（disease-free survival，DFS）[2]。MAC 预处理中清髓剂量药物具有较强毒性，推荐用于患者年龄≤60 岁且不伴重要脏器功能受损或移植合并症指数较低（HCT-CI<3）的各类白血病患者。

AML 移植经典 MAC 预处理方案包含含全身放疗的 Cy/TBI 方案[CTX 60mg/（kg·d）×2 +TBI 10~13.5Gy]和化疗为主的 BU/Cy 方案[静脉注射 BU 剂量 3.2mg/（kg·d）×4 或口服 BU 剂量 4mg/（kg·d）×4+Cy 60mg/（kg·d）×2][3]。BU 首先推荐静脉注射制剂（iv-Bu），避免口服 BU 药代动力学个体差异大和呕吐导致给药剂量不足等问题，降低移植后肝窦阻塞综合征（SINusoidal obstruction syndrome，SOS）及相关非复发死亡（non-relapse mortality，NRM）[4]。AML 接受 Cy/TBI 和 iv-Bu/Cy 预处理无病生存期（leukemia-free survival，LFS）和总生存期（overall survival，OS）差异无统计学意义[5]。改良 Bu/Cy 方案组成为阿糖胞苷[Cytarabine，4g/（m²·d）×2 + BU 3.2mg/（kg·d）×3 + Cy 1.8g/（m²·d）×2]+ 司莫司汀[Semustine，250mg/（m²·d）×1]。改良 Bu/Cy 方案在中国临床应用广泛，适用于不同供体移植包括 HLA 相合同胞供体、非血缘供体和 HLA 不相合亲缘供体[6]。Flu/Bu 方案组成为 Flu 30mg/（m²·d）×5+Bu 3.2mg/（kg·d）×4。Flu/Bu 移植方案与 Bu/Cy 随机对照研究结果差异无统计学意义[7]。对于 40~65 岁 AML 患者，Flu/Bu 预处理较经典 Bu/Cy 的 NRM 更低[8]。

ALL 移植经典 MAC 预处理以 Cy/TBI 为主，Cy/TBI 方案与口服 Bu/Cy 比较，早期毒性反应（如 SOS）低，复发率低，显著提高 OS。在<35 岁年轻成人 ALL 移植 Cy/TBI 与 iv-Bu/Cy 比较，能显著降低复发率，尤其 CR2 期或进展期移植病例，并提高 LFS 和 OS[9]。大剂量 Vp-16（900~1 800mg/m^2）可替代 Cy 与 TBI 联合组成 Vp/TBI 方案。EBMT 数据库回顾性分析提示 Vp/TBI 显著降低 Ph-ALL 移植后复发，提高 LFS 和无复发/无 GVHD 生存期（GVHD and relapse free survival，GRFS）[10]。新近研究表明化疗预处理方案 iv-Bu/Cy 预处理与 Cy/TBI（9gy）差异无统计学意义，iv-Bu/Cy，推荐作为无法接受 TBI 患者的替代方案[8, 11]。改良 Bu/CY 方案则适用于 ALL，包括 Ph+ALL[6]。近年来，新型靶向治疗药物如低甲基化药物等与清髓预处理联合，有可能进一步提高标准预处理方案的疗效[12]。

4.2 减低毒性（RTC）、降低强度（RIC）或非清髓（NMA）预处理

	Ⅰ级推荐	Ⅱ级推荐	Ⅲ级推荐
RTC/RIC	含全身放疗预处理： 　Flu/TBI（8Gy）（2A 类）		
	化疗预处理： 　Flu/Bu（3d）（2A 类） 　Flu/Mel（2A 类）		TBF（2B 类） MBF（3 类）

减低毒性（RTC）、降低强度（RIC）或非清髓（NMA）预处理（续）

	I级推荐	II级推荐	III级推荐
NMA	含全身放疗预处理： Flu/TBI（2Gy）（2A类）		Flu/Treo/TBI（2Gy）（3类）
	化疗预处理： Flu/BU（1~2d）（2A类）	Flu/Treo （I B类）	Flu/Cy（3类）

注：TBF. 塞替派（thiothepa, T）+白消安（busulfan, B）+福达拉滨（fludarabine, F）；Treo. 苏消安（treosulfan）。BMF. 美法仑（melphalan, M）+白消安（busulfan, B）+福达拉滨（fludarabine, F）

【注释】

随着对移植物抗白血病效应（graft versus leukemia, GVL）认识和研究，新型移植预处理方案不断出现，其主要特点是预处理放疗和化疗强度减低，不完全具备清除宿主骨髓造血功能作用。通过增强预处理清除宿主免疫作用保证供体细胞植入，并在移植后诱导 GVL 效应达到治愈白血病目的。放/化疗药物的非清髓性剂量定义为 TBI $\leq$ 5Gy；BU 总量 $\leq$ 9mg/kg；美法仑（melphalan, Mel）$\leq$ 140mg/m^2、塞替派（thiothepa, Thio）$\leq$ 10mg/kg。减低预处理根据清除骨髓造血强度分为非清髓移植（non-myeloablative regimen, NMA）、减低强度预处理（reduced-intensity conditioning, RIC）或减低毒性预处理（reduced toxicity conditioning, RTC），如 Flu/Bu 方案中 iv-BU 3.2mg/（kg·d）给药 1~2 天为 NMA，3 天为 RTC，目前倾向于统一称"减低强度预处理（RIC）"。

RIC 方案优势在于降低预处理强度，减轻移植预处理毒性及相关 NRM，适用于无法耐受标准 MAC 预处理的髓系白血病患者（AML/MDS/CML）如年龄>60 岁或年龄≤60 岁伴重要脏器功能受损或 HCT-CI 积分≥3。ALL 接受 RIC 预处理复发率相对较高，临床较少采用。

对于 AML 病例，CIBMTR 数据提示 DRI 高危或极高危患者 MAC 和 RIC 移植预处理疗效总体相当，DFS 和 OS 差异无统计学意义[2]。随机对照研究证实 RIC 与 MAC 方案治疗 AML 和 MDS 患者整体 NRM，复发率，DFS 和 OS 均差异无统计学意义[13-15]。

经典RIC方案保留中等强度TBI 和/或烷化剂药物（如BU或Mel）。包括含全身放疗Flu/TBI（8）方案：Flu 30mg/（m²·d）× 5 + TBI 8Gy[16]。化疗预处理方案包括Flu/Bu（3）方案［Flu 50mg/（m²·d）× 5+Bu 3.2mg/（kg·d）× 3 或在此基础上增加阿糖胞苷等抗白血病药物］和Flu/Mel（140）方案（Flu 150mg/m² + Mel 40mg/m²）。系统分析（meta analysis）多项随机对照临床研究结果提示 RIC 预处理长期疗效与清髓性预处理无显著差异。

减低剂量预处理还包括新型预处理药物如苏消安（treosulfan）和塞替派（thiotepa）。苏消安暂无清髓性强度明确定义，Flu 和苏消安为主的 Flu/Treo 方案（Flu 150mg/m² + Treo 36~42mg/m²）暂时认定为 RIC 方案。随机对照研究提示在 AML/MDS 移植中 Flu/Treo 方案非劣于/优于经典 Flu/Bu（2）方案[17]。含塞替派的 TBF 方案［thiotepa 5mg/（kg·d）× 2 + Flu 50mg/（m²·d）× 5+BU 130mg/（m²·d）×（2~3）］与Flu/Bu4方案移植后整体疗效相当。含美法仑和白消安的双烷化剂预处理MBF［M 50~70mg/（m²·d）× 2 + BU 6.4mg/（kg·d）× 2+ Flu 30mg/（m²·d）× 5］具有较低的复发率和可控的 NRM[18]。

经典 NMA 方案以含全身放疗的方案 Flu/TBI 为主［Flu 30mg/（m²·d）× 5 + TBI 2Gy］和化疗为主的 Flu/Bu（Bu 1~2 天）。随机对照研究提示 Flu/TBI 与 Flu/Bu（2）比较，移植后早期毒性反应和 NRM 明显减低,但复发率增高,总体 OS 和 LFS 无显著差异。化疗预处理方案还包括 Flu/Cy(Flu 150mg/m^2 + Cy 120~140mg/kg)等。

4.3 增强预处理和强化疗序贯移植预处理

	Ⅰ级推荐	Ⅱ级推荐	Ⅲ级推荐
强化预处理	含全身放疗预处理		Vp/Cy/TBI(ALL,2B 类) Vp/Cy/TBI(AML,3 类)
	化疗预处理	地西他滨-By/Cy (MDS/sAML,1B 类)	Bu/Cy/IDA(3 类)
强化疗序贯移植预处理	含全身放疗预处理		FLAMSA-Flu/TBI(2Gy)(2A 类) Flu/Treo/TBI(2Gy)(3 类)
	化疗预处理		FLAMSA-Flu/BU(2A 类) CA-Flu/Bu(3 类) Mel-Flu/Treo(3 类) TCE-Flu/Bu(3 类) FLAG-IDA/CLAGE-Flu/Bu(3 类) CLAGM-Bu/Cy(3 类)

注:IDA. 去甲氧柔红霉素(idarubicin);FLAMSA. Flu + 阿糖胞苷(Ara-C)+ 安吖啶(amsacrine,AMSA);CA. 氯法拉滨(clofarabine)+ 阿糖胞苷(Ara-C);TCE. thiotepa + Cy + VP-16。

【注释】

对于高危或复发 AML/ALL，常规 MAC 预处理移植后仍有较高复发率，因此在清髓预处理基础上联合具有较强抗白血病作用药物如去甲氧柔红霉素或依托泊苷，可增强移植治疗的抗白血病作用，但也增加移植后早期毒性反应和相关 NRM。推荐用于相对年轻且不伴重要脏器受损和 HCT-CI 高风险人群。MAC 预处理 Cy-TBI 中加入中-大剂量依托泊苷（VP-16 30~40mg/kg）治疗高危 ALL 如第一次缓解期（CR1）骨髓微小残留白血病（measurable residual disease，MRD）阳性或伴高危细胞核型异常或第二次缓解期（CR2），显著降低移植后复发且不增加移植后 NRM[19]。新近在儿童 ALL 移植治疗的随机对照研究提示 VP-16/TBI 优于化疗预处理[20]。Bu/Cy 方案加入大剂量去甲氧柔红霉素[15mg/（m²·d）×3]能提高 MRD+AML/ALL 移植后疗效。对于高危 MDS 和 MDS 转化 sAML，Bu/CY 方案加入地西他滨显著降低移植后复发，未显著增加移植后 NRM，提高移植后生存[21]。

对于初治未缓解或难治性 AML 移植前给予大剂量化疗降低白血病负荷，化疗结束后间隔 3~7 天或直接序贯不同强度移植预处理，能获得较高完全缓解率，2 年 OS 和 DFS 可达 30%~50%[22-25]。FLAMSA 化疗[Flu 30mg/（m²·d）×5 + Ara-C 2g/（m²·d）×4 + AMSA 100mg/（m²·d）×4]间隔 3 天序贯 RIC 方案 Cy/TBI（Cy 80~120mg/kg + TBI 4Gy）方案对于初治未缓解 AML 预期 OS~60%[22]。45~65 岁 CR1/CR2 期高危成人 AML 患者，FLASMA 序贯 RIC 预处理方案同样具有较好疗效，与 Flu-Treo 为主预处理比较显著降低移植后复发，提高 RFS，但国内 AMSA 存在药物可及性问题。TCE[Thiotepa 5mg/（kg·d）×2 + Cy 400mg/（m²·d）×4 + VP-16 100mg/（m²·d）×4]或 CA[Clofarabine 30mg/（m²·d）×5 + Ara-C 1g/（m²·d）×5]方案序贯降低强度 Flu/Bu 或 Bu/Cy 预处理治疗难治恶性血液病具有一定疗效。FLAG-IDA 或 CLAGM 是复发 AML 的再诱导方案，序贯 iv-Bu 为主预处理

治疗难治性 AML 均获得较高缓解率，2 年 OS/DFS 达到 40%~50%[23-24]。未缓解或难治性 ALL 强烈化疗序贯预处理方案未获得较满意疗效，临床不推荐应用[25]。

4.4 重度再生障碍性贫血（SAA）移植预处理

	Ⅰ级推荐	Ⅱ级推荐	Ⅲ级推荐
不含全身放疗预处理	CTX 200mg/kg -rATG 10mg/kg		Flu 120mg/m^2 + CY 120~200mg/kg+ rATG 10mg/kg （2B 类） IV-BU 6.4mg/kg + Cy 200mg/kg + rATG 10mg/kg （2B 类）
含全身放疗预处理			rATG 4.5mg/kg + Flu 150mg/m^2 + CY 14.5mg/kg×2 + TBI 2Gy（2B 类） Flu（120~200mg/m^2）+ Cy（120~200mg/kg）+ rATG 10mg/kg 或 ATG-F 20~30mg/kg + TBI 3Gy （2B 类）

注：rATG. 兔抗人胸腺球蛋白；ATG-F. ATG-Fresenius。

【注释】

急性重症再生障碍性贫血（severe aplastic anemia，SAA）造血干细胞移植与经典的免疫抑制治疗比较可获得持久的血液学反应和更低的复发率，尤其是同胞全合供者骨髓移植作为成人 SAA 的首选治疗。SAA 移植治疗预处理以充分的免疫抑制为主要目的，以大剂量环磷酰胺和兔抗胸腺球蛋白（rATG）为主。对于植入失败率相对较高的移植类型如非血缘供体和单倍体供者移植，则给予强化免疫抑制方案，在 Cy-ATG 基础上增加 fludarabine 或 BU 或小剂量 TBI 以保证植入[26-27]。

参考文献

[1] SCOTT BL, PASQUINI MC, LOGAN BR, et al. Myeloablative versus reduced-intensity hematopoietic cell transplantation for acute myeloid leukemia and myelodysplastic syndromes. J Clin Oncol, 2017, 35 (11): 1154-1161.

[2] BEJANYAN N, ZHANG M, BO-SUBAIT K, et al. Myeloablative conditioning for allogeneic transplantation results in superior disease-free survival for acute myelogenous leukemia and myelodysplastic syndromes with low/intermediate but not high disease risk index: A center for international blood and marrow transplant research study. Transplant Cell Ther, 2021, 27 (1): 68.

[3] SOCIÉ G, CLIFT RA, BLAISE D, et al. Busulfan plus cyclophosphamide compared with total-body irradiation plus cyclophosphamide before marrow transplantation for myeloid leukemia: Long-term follow-up of 4 randomized studies. Blood, 2001, 98 (13): 3569-3574.

[4] KASHYAP A, WINGARD J, CAGNONI P, et al. Intravenous versus oral busulfan as part of a busulfan/cyclophosphamide preparative regimen for allogeneic hematopoietic stem cell transplantation: Decreased incidence of hepatic

venoocclusive disease (HVOD), HVOD-related mortality, and overall 100-day mortality. Biol Blood Marrow Transplant, 2002, 8 (9): 493-500.
[5] NAGLER A, ROCHA V, LABOPIN M, et al. Allogeneic hematopoietic stem-cell transplantation for acute myeloid leukemia in remission: comparison of intravenous busulfan plus cyclophosphamide (Cy) versus total-body irradiation plus Cy as conditioning regimen: A report from the acute leukemia working party of the European group for blood and marrow transplantation. J Clin Oncol, 2013, 31 (28): 3549-3556.
[6] HUANG XJ, LIU DH, LIU KY, et al. Treatment of acute leukemia with unmanipulated HLA-mismatched/haploidentical blood and bone marrow transplantation. Biol Blood Marrow Transplant, 2009, 15 (2): 257-265.
[7] LIU H, ZHAI X, SONG Z, et al. Busulfan plus fludarabine as a myeloablative conditioning regimen compared with busulfan plus cyclophosphamide for acute myeloid leukemia in first complete remission undergoing allogeneic hematopoietic stem cell transplantation: A prospective and multicenter study. J Hematol Oncol, 2013, 6: 15.
[8] RAMBALDI A, GRASSI A, MASCIULLI A, et al. Busulfan plus cyclophosphamide versus busulfan plus fludarabine as a preparative regimen for allogeneic haemopoietic stem-cell transplantation in patients with acute myeloid leukaemia: An open-label, multicentre, randomised, phase 3 trial. Lancet Oncol, 2015, 16 (15): 1525-1536.
[9] CAHU X, LABOPIN M, GIEBEL S, et al. Impact of conditioning with TBI in adult patients with T-cell ALL who receive a myeloablative allogeneic stem cell transplantation: A report from the acute leukemia working party of EBMT. Bone Marrow Transplant, 2016, 51 (3): 351-357.
[10] CZYZ A, LABOPIN M, GIEBEL S, et al. Cyclophosphamide versus etoposide in combination with total body irradiation as conditioning regimen for adult patients with Ph-negative acute lymphoblastic leukemia undergoing allogeneic stem cell transplant: On behalf of the ALWP of the European Society for Blood and Marrow Transplantation. Am J Hematol, 2018, 93 (6): 778-785.
[11] ZHANG H, FAN Z, HUANG F, et al. Busulfan plus cyclophosphamide versus total body irradiation plus cyclo-

phosphamide for adults acute b lymphoblastic leukemia: An open-label, multicenter, phase Ⅲ trial. J Clin Oncol, 2023, 10; 41 (2): 343-353.

[12] TANG X, VALDEZ BC, MA Y, et al. Low-dose decitabine as part of a modified Bu-Cy conditioning regimen improves survival in AML patients with active disease undergoing allogeneic hematopoietic stem cell transplantation. Bone Marrow Transplant, 2021, 56 (7): 1674-1682.

[13] BORNHÄUSER M, KIENAST J, TRENSCHEL R, et al. Reduced-intensity conditioning versus standard conditioning before allogeneic haemopoietic cell transplantation in patients with acute myeloid leukaemia in first complete remission: A prospective, open-label randomised phase 3 trial. Lancet Oncol, 2012, 13 (10): 1035-1044.

[14] KRÖGER N, IACOBELLI S, FRANKE GN, et al. Dose-reduced versus standard conditioning followed by allogeneic stem-cell transplantation for patients with myelodysplastic syndrome: A prospective randomized phase Ⅲ study of the EBMT (RICMAC Trial). J Clin Oncol, 2017, 35 (19): 2157-2164.

[15] SCOTT BL. Long-term follow up of BMT CTN 0901, a randomized phase Ⅲ trial comparing myeloablative (MAC) to reduced intensity conditioning (RIC) prior to hematopoietic cell transplantation (HCT) for acute myeloid leukemia (AML) or myelodysplasia (MDS)(MAC vs. RIC Trial). Biol Blood Marrow Transplant, 2020, 26: S11.

[16] BEELEN DW, TRENSCHEL R, STELLJES M, et al. Treosulfan or busulfan plus fludarabine as conditioning treatment before allogeneic haemopoietic stem cell transplantation for older patients with acute myeloid leukaemia or myelodysplastic syndrome (MC-FludT. 14/L): A randomised, non-inferiority, phase 3 trial. Lancet Haematol, 2020, 7 (1): e28-e39.

[17] RINGDÉN O, ERKERS T, ASCHAN J, et al. A prospective randomized toxicity study to compare reduced-intensity and myeloablative conditioning in patients with myeloid leukaemia undergoing allogeneic haematopoietic stem cell transplantation. J Intern Med, 2013, 274 (2): 153-162.

[18] JIANG JL, CHEN M, WANG LN, et al. Double alkylators based conditioning reduced the relapse rate after allogeneic peripheral blood stem cell transplantation in adult patients with myeloid malignancies: A single arm phase Ⅱ study. Bone Marrow Transplant, 2022, 57 (5): 843-845.

[19] ARAI Y, KONDO T, SHIGEMATSU A, et al. Improved prognosis with additional medium-dose VP16 to CY/TBI in allogeneic transplantation for high risk ALL in adults. Am J Hematol, 2018, 93 (1): 47-57.

[20] PETERS C, DALLE JH, LOCATELLI F, et al. Total body irradiation or chemotherapy conditioning in childhood ALL: A multinational, randomized, noninferiority phase Ⅲ study. J Clin Oncol, 2021, 39 (4): 295-307.

[21] XUAN L, DAI M, JIANG E, et al. The effect of granulocyte-colony stimulating factor, decitabine, and busulfan-cyclophosphamide versus busulfan-cyclophosphamide conditioning on relapse in patients with myelodysplastic syndrome or secondary acute myeloid leukaemia evolving from myelodysplastic syndrome undergoing allogeneic haematopoietic stem-cell transplantation: An open-label, multicentre, randomised, phase 3 trial. Lancet Haematol, 2023: S2352-3026 (22) 00375-1.

[22] SCHMID C, SCHLEUNING M, SCHWERDTFEGER R, et al. Long-term survival in refractory acute myeloid leukemia after sequential treatment with chemotherapy and reduced-intensity conditioning for allogeneic stem cell transplantation. Blood, 2006, 108 (3): 1092-1099.

[23] WANG L, DEVILLIER R, WAN M, et al. Clinical outcome of FLAG-IDA chemotherapy sequential with Flu-Bu3 conditioning regimen in patients with refractory AML: A parallel study from Shanghai Institute of Hematology and Institut Paoli-Calmettes. Bone Marrow Transplant, 2019, 54 (3): 458-464.

[24] XIAO H, LI L, PANG Y, et al. Sequential treatment combining cladribine-based re-induction, myeloablative allogeneic HSCT, and prophylactic donor lymphocyte infusion: A promising treatment for refractory acute myeloid leukemia. Ann Hematol, 2018, 97 (12): 2479-2490.

[25] BAZARBACHI AH, AL HAMED R, LABOPIN M, et al. Allogeneic stem-cell transplantation with sequential con-

ditioning in adult patients with refractory or relapsed acute lymphoblastic leukemia: A report from the EBMT Acute Leukemia Working Party. Bone Marrow Transplant, 2020, 55 (3): 595-602.
[26] IFTIKHAR R, CHAUDHRY Q, ANWER F, et al. Allogeneic hematopoietic stem cell transplantation in aplastic anemia: Current indications and transplant strategies. Blood Rev, 2021, 47: 100772.
[27] ZHANG XH, CHEN J, HAN MZ, et al. The consensus from The Chinese Society of Hematology on indications, conditioning regimens and donor selection for allogeneic hematopoietic stem cell transplantation: 2021 update. J Hematol Oncol, 2021, 14: 145-164.

5 异基因造血干细胞移植供者动员、细胞采集及回输

	Ⅰ级推荐	Ⅱ级推荐	Ⅲ级推荐
动员剂	G-CSF（2A 类）		
外周血干细胞采集	采集时间：G-CSF 动员 4~5 天时采集 采集数量：CD34+ 细胞数 $\geqslant 2 \times 10^6$/kg [a]，单个核细胞数 $\geqslant 5 \times 10^8$/kg [a]	对复发高危倾向的患者，建议预先采集出后续治疗所需的细胞冻存	
骨髓血采集			采集细胞数量：有核细胞数 $\geqslant 2 \times 10^8$/kg [a]

异基因造血干细胞移植供者动员、细胞采集及回输（续）

	I 级推荐	II 级推荐	III 级推荐
回输	血型不合： 外周血干细胞：直接回输 b 骨髓血：供受者血型主侧不合需进行去红处理 次侧不合根据抗体效价选择去浆处理 主次侧不合选择去红去浆处理		

注：a. 为建议细胞阈值，临床实践中少于上述阈值也可能获得异体植入；b. 采集中要注意避免混入大量红细胞。

【注释】

外周血干细胞是目前异基因造血干细胞移植最常用的干细胞来源。粒细胞刺激因子（G-CSF）是被最广泛采用的干细胞动员剂，常用剂量是 5~10μg/（kg·d）。在该剂量范围内 G-CSF 的剂量与外周血 $CD34^+$ 细胞数的增长呈正相关[1-4]。更高剂量的 G-CSF（12μg/kg，2 次/d）可以在更短的时间内获得更高的采集数量[5]，但骨痛、乏力头疼等副作用更多、费用更高，出于对供者安全考虑一般不予推荐。也有小样本的报道应用粒细胞巨噬细胞刺激因子（GM-CSF）、长效 G-CSF 和新型动员剂普乐沙福（plerixafor）进行动员取得了成功，但所有这些都缺乏足够证据证明优于 G-CSF，目前也没有在临床广泛应用,故未写入指南推荐。粒细胞数量在应用 G-CSF 后 5 天达到高峰,而 CD34$^+$ 细胞的峰值一般在动员后 4~6 天达到,所以推荐在 G-CSF 动员后 4~5 天开始采集干细胞[6]。

目前仍无法确定保证异体植入的最低干细胞阈值,一般移植中心规定的可接受的 CD34$^+$ 细胞阈值是 2×10^6/kg,静态骨髓有核细胞数是 2×10^8/kg。当然输注少于上述数值的干细胞也可能获得异体植入,但往往伴随植入延迟和/或植入不良。而更多的干细胞意味着更快的造血植入和更低的感染发生率,复发率以及非复发死亡率(NRM),但也有可能增加 GVHD 的风险[7-11]。因此,一般推荐 CD34+ 细胞数为($4~5$)$\times 10^6$/kg,不超过 8×10^6/kg[4]。

静态骨髓干细胞目前在临床应用越来越少,但在再生障碍性贫血和儿童患者移植中有优势[12-15]。随着单倍体移植的进展,部分中心采用经 G-CSF 动员的骨髓干细胞和外周血干细胞混合移植的模式[16-18]。具体选用哪种干细胞,需要各中心根据各自经验、规范和患者的疾病类型、分期阶段,以及供受者身体条件等综合决定。

参考文献

[1] DREGER P, HAFERLACH T, ECKSTEIN V, et al. G-CSF-mobilized peripheral blood progenitor cells for allogeneic transplantation: Safety, kinetics of mobilization, and composition of the graft. Br J Haematol, 1994, 87 (3): 609-613.

[2] FISCHMEISTER G, KURZ M, HAAS OA, et al. G-CSF versus GM-CSF for stimulation of peripheral blood progenitor cells (PBPC) and leukocytes in healthy volunteers: Comparison of efficacy and tolerability. Ann Hematol, 1999, 78 (3): 117-123.

[3] ANDERLINI P, DONATO M, CHAN KW, et al. Allogeneic blood progenitor cell collection in normal donors after mobilization with filgrastim: the M. D. Anderson Cancer Center experience. Transfusion, 1999, 39 (6): 555-560.

[4] DUONG HK, SAVANI BN, COPELAN E, et al. Peripheral blood progenitor cell mobilization for autologous and allogeneic hematopoietic cell transplantation: Guidelines from the American Society for Blood and Marrow Transplantation. Biol Blood Marrow Transplant, 2014, 20 (9): 1262-1273.

[5] ENGELHARDT M, BERTZ H, AFTING M, et al. High-versus standard-dose filgrastim (rhG-CSF) for mobilization of peripheral-blood progenitor cells from allogeneic donors and CD34 (+) immunoselection. J Clin Oncol, 1999, 17 (7): 2160-2172.

[6] GRIGG AP, ROBERTS AW, RAUNOW H, et al. Optimizing dose and scheduling of filgrastim (granulocyte colony-stimulating factor) for mobilization and collection of peripheral blood progenitor cells in normal volunteers. Blood, 1995, 86 (12): 4437-4445.

[7] GORIN NC, LABOPIN M, BOIRON JM, et al. Results of genoidentical hemopoietic stem cell transplantation with reduced intensity conditioning for acute myelocytic leukemia: Higher doses of stem cells infused benefit patients receiving transplants in second remission or beyond: The Acute Leukemia Working Party of the European Cooperative Group for Blood and Marrow Transplantation. J Clin Oncol, 2006, 24 (24): 3959-3966.

[8] NAKAMURA R, AUAYPORN N, SMITH DD, et al. Impact of graft cell dose on transplant outcomes following unrelated donor allogeneic peripheral blood stem cell transplantation: Higher CD34+ cell doses are associated with decreased relapse rates. Biol Blood Marrow Transplant, 2008, 14 (4): 449-457.

[9] ISLAM MS, ANOOP P, DATTA-NEMDHARRY P, et al. Implications of CD34+ cell dose on clinical and haematological outcome of allo-SCT for acquired aplastic anaemia. Bone Marrow Transplant, 2010, 45 (5): 886-894.

[10] ZAUCHA JM, GOOLEY T, BENSINGER WI, et al. CD34 cell dose in granulocyte colony-stimulating factor-mobilized peripheral blood mononuclear cell grafts affects engraftment kinetics and development of extensive chronic graft-versus-

host disease after human leukocyte antigen-identical sibling transplantation. Blood, 2001, 98 (12): 3221-3227.
[11] MOHTY M, BILGER K, JOURDAN E, et al. Higher doses of CD34+ peripheral blood stem cells are associated with increased mortality from chronic graft-versus-host disease after allogeneic HLA-identical sibling transplantation. Leukemia, 2003, 17 (5): 869-875.
[12] SIMONIN M, DALISSIER A, LABOPIN M, et al. More chronic GvHD and non-relapse mortality after peripheral blood stem cell compared with bone marrow in hematopoietic transplantation for paediatric acute lymphoblastic leukemia: A retrospective study on behalf of the EBMT Paediatric Diseases Working Party. Bone Marrow Transplant, 2017, 52 (7): 1071-1073.
[13] BACIGALUPO A, SOCIÉ G, SCHREZENMEIER H, et al. Bone marrow versus peripheral blood as the stem cell source for sibling transplants in acquired aplastic anemia: Survival advantage for bone marrow in all age groups. Haematologica, 2012, 97 (8): 1142-1148.
[14] EAPEN M, LE RADEMACHER J, ANTIN JH, et al. Effect of stem cell source on outcomes after unrelated donor transplantation in severe aplastic anemia. Blood, 2011, 118 (9): 2618-2621.
[15] BHELLA S, MAJHAIL NS, BETCHER J, et al. Choosing wisely BMT: American Society for Blood and Marrow Transplantation and Canadian Blood and Marrow Transplant Group's List of 5 tests and treatments to question in blood and marrow transplantation. Biol Blood Marrow Transplant, 2018, 24 (5): 909-913.
[16] HUANG XJ, LIU DH, LIU KY, et al. Haploidentical hematopoietic stem cell transplantation without in vitro T-cell depletion for the treatment of hematological malignancies. Bone Marrow Transplant, 2006, 38 (4): 291-297.
[17] WANG Y, LIU QF, XU LP, et al. Haploidentical vs identical-sibling transplant for AML in remission: A multicenter, prospective study. Blood, 2015, 125 (25): 3956-3962.
[18] KASAMON YL, AMBINDER RF, FUCHS EJ, et al. Prospective study of nonmyeloablative, HLA-mismatched unrelated BMT with high-dose posttransplantation cyclophosphamide. Blood Adv, 2017, 1 (4): 288-292.

6 异基因造血干细胞移植后急性移植物抗宿主病的预防、诊断及治疗

6.1 急性移植物抗宿主病预防药物推荐

		Ⅰ级推荐	Ⅱ级推荐	Ⅲ级推荐
不同供者来源移植体系 aGVHD 预防	同胞全合	钙调磷酸酶抑制剂联合一种抗代谢药物霉酚酸酯（MMF）或 MTX（1A 类）	选择他克莫司（FK506）或者环孢素（CsA），可以按照移植中心的用药经验（1B 类）；兔抗胸腺细胞球蛋白（rATG）（1B 类）	
	无关供者	rATG（1A 类）	钙调磷酸酶抑制剂联合一种抗代谢药物（MMF 或 MTX）；选择 FK506 或者 CsA 可以按照移植中心的用药经验（1B 类）	
	单倍体相合	rATG（1A 类）；钙调磷酸酶抑制剂联合二种抗代谢药物（MMF 与 MTX）	FK506 或者 CsA 均可以按照移植中心的用药经验（1B 类）；在重度口腔黏膜炎患者，+11 天 MTX 可不用（2A 类）	
	脐带血		CsA 联合 MMF（1B 类）	rATG（2B 类）

急性移植物抗宿主病预防药物推荐（续）

		I 级推荐	II 级推荐	III 级推荐
不同预处理强度移植体系 aGVHD 预防	清髓性	推荐钙调蛋白抑制剂联合 MTX（1A 类）	MMF 可以替代 MTX 用于不适合应用 MTX 或需要快速植入（2A 类）	
	非清髓或者减毒预处理方案	推荐钙调蛋白抑制剂（1A 类）	抗代谢药物推荐使用 MMF 代替 MTX（2A 类）	
供者淋巴细胞回输（DLI）后 aGVHD 预防	干预性或者治疗性 DLI		DLI 后是否需要短程免疫抑制治疗，需根据回输时间、剂量、GVHD 发生情况等因素综合考虑	DLI 时将 CsA 调整至有效浓度。也可以单用 MTX 预防
	预防性 DLI		DLI 后是否需要短程免疫抑制治疗，需根据回输时间、剂量、GVHD 发生情况等因素综合考虑	DLI 时将 CsA 调整至有效浓度。也可以单用 MTX 预防

【注释】

目前 ATG 在异基因造血干细胞移植中得到广泛应用,单倍体相合、无关供者及同胞全合移植中,多个高质量前瞻随机对照研究均证实,ATG 可以明显降低急慢性移植物抗宿主病(GVHD)的发生[1-8]。

环孢素联合 MTX 与 FK506 联合 MTX 相比,两者在控制 GVHD 及总生存方面疗效类似[8-9]。多数移植中心可能更习惯应用 CsA。清髓性移植中,钙调磷酸酶抑制剂联合 MTX 预防 GVHD 的疗效已经得到证实。meta 分析及回顾性研究显示,与钙调磷酸酶抑制剂联合 MMF 相比,钙调磷酸酶抑制剂联合 MTX 能够明显降低 Ⅲ~Ⅳ度 aGVHD 的发生,Ⅱ~Ⅳ度 aGVHD 发生率两者类似。非清髓或者 RIC 方案移植中,MMF 优于 MTX 的证据级别较低。在单倍体相合移植中,MMF 推荐 +1 个月剂量减半,可以用到 +2 个月。MMF 应用时间根据复发风险和 GVHD 情况调整,在无 GVHD 的高复发风险患者或病毒感染的患者,可提前停用 MMF(2A 类)。近年针对 GVHD 高危患者开展一些探索,如在 haplo-HSCT 中以生物标记(骨髓移植物的 CD4 细胞/CD8 细胞比值)为指导分层短期应用低剂量糖皮质激素、在母系或旁系 HID-HSCT 后加用低剂量环磷酰胺,均能有效降低 aGVHD 发生率[2, 8]。

既往脐带血造血干细胞移植多用 ATG,近年有学者认为 UCBT 不用 ATG 也是可行的[10]。孙自敏等报告采用全身放疗的清髓性预处理方案进行 UCBT,预防 GVHD 采用环孢素联合 MMF,对照组为基于白消安的清髓预处理 CBT,采用 CsA+MMF+MTX 或 ATG[fresenius,7.5mg/(kg·d)×3d]预防 GVHD,结果显示两组间 Ⅱ~Ⅳ、Ⅲ~Ⅳ度 aGVHD 的发生率差异均无统计学意义,GRFS 也差异无统计学意义。

DLI 后是否需要短程免疫抑制治疗，需根据回输时间、剂量、GVHD 发生情况等因素综合考虑。北京大学人民医院报道 CsA 在 DLI 前 1 天开始应用，并调整至有效浓度范围，持续时间因不同移植类型而异，建议同胞全合移植患者 DLI 后 4~6 周减停，单倍体相合移植患者 DLI 后 6~8 周减停。干预性 DLI 后预防 GVHD 也可以单用 MTX，+1、+4、+8 天，以后每周 10mg 口服，共 4~6 周（2B 类）。

6.2 急性移植物抗宿主病预防药物用药方法推荐

	Ⅰ级推荐	Ⅱ级推荐	Ⅲ级推荐
环孢素（CsA）		CsA 移植后第 1 周建议谷浓度 200~300μg/L（2A 类） 检测抽血时间建议用药后 12 小时（2A 类） 标准 CsA 预防同胞全合使用时长为 6 个月，单倍体和非血缘供者为 6~9 个月（2A 类） 再生障碍性贫血患者至少 9~12 个月，减量至停用的时间至少 3 个月以上（2A 类） 除非存在轻度皮肤 aGVHD，如果存在 aGVHD 或者 cGVHD 征象，CsA 一般不考虑减量。在疾病复发进展状态且没有 GVHD 情况下，CsA 可以谨慎减量（2A 类）	CsA 回输前开始使用，每天两次或者 24 小时持续输注，建议起始剂量 3mg/（kg·d）（2B 类） 大部分患者移植后 3 个月内目标浓度 100~200μg/L（2C 类） 临床实际操作中，需要根据疾病复发、嵌合状态及 GVHD 等因素统筹考虑（2C 类）

急性移植物抗宿主病预防药物用药方法推荐(续)

	I级推荐	II级推荐	III级推荐
MTX		清髓性移植患者中，MTX的初始剂量为15mg/(m^2·d)，移植后第1天使用 +3天、+6天、+11天继续应用MTX，剂量为10mg/(m^2·d)（2A类） 亚叶酸钙解救治疗通常在MTX使用后的24小时应用（2A类）	
MMF		静脉或者口服，10~15mg/kg，每天用2~3次，根据毒性调整剂量（2A类） 通常移植后+1天开始应用，预防方案通常在同胞全合中持续30天，无关供者移植中应用2~3个月	使用时间可以根据疾病复发风险和GVHD风险来调整，例如可以根据供受者性别和回输的T淋巴细胞来调整，如果疾病处于进展或者复发状态，MMF可以考虑提前停用（2B类）
rATG		多应用rATG，同胞全合移植中推荐用量为4.5mg/(kg·d)，无关供者移植和单倍体移植推荐用量为7.5~10mg/(kg·d)；更高的剂量与高感染风险相关（2A类） 再生障碍性贫血患者推荐使用ATG，具体用量根据预处理方案中环磷酰胺、TBI是否使用等因素调整（2A类）	也可应用ATG-F或ATG-P

【注释】

aGVHD 预防药物推荐的证据级别普遍较低,缺乏较好的前瞻随机对照性研究,证据主要来自专家共识和实际使用经验。回顾性研究证实,回输后 1 周内 CsA 浓度维持 200~300μg/L,能够明显降低 aGVHD 发生[11]。临床实践中,CsA 浓度调整需要根据疾病复发、嵌合体及 GVHD 等因素统筹考虑。

钙调磷酸酶抑制剂及 MMF 减量的方法也是争议比较大的地方[12-13]。有报道,标危白血病患者异基因造血干细胞移植后,CsA 于移植后 6 个月全部减停的患者总体生存率较高,高危白血病患者钙调磷酸酶抑制剂更早时间减停(有报道 2 个月)也许可以改善预后[12]。因此,本指南推荐白血病标危患者同胞全合移植后 6 个月减停钙调磷酸酶抑制剂。减剂量预处理方案中,移植后 +3 天、+6 天通常使用更低剂量的 MTX。ATG 在不同移植背景下的使用剂量、使用时长及剂型,目前还没有定论[3-5]。同胞全合移植中 rATG 用量 2.5~5mg/kg 也可以应用。再生障碍性贫血患者 ATG 用量范围较大,具体用量根据预处理方案中环磷酰胺、TBI 是否使用、移植类型等因素调整[14-15],例如同胞全合移植单用环磷酰胺预处理方案中 rATG 推荐 10~20mg/kg,同胞全合移植中氟达拉滨联合环磷酰胺预处理方案 rATG 推荐 5~20mg/kg,北京大学人民医院报道单倍体移植中 rATG 推荐 10mg/kg。

6.3 急性移植物抗宿主病诊断及分度标准

		Ⅰ级推荐	Ⅱ级推荐	Ⅲ级推荐
诊断标准	临床诊断	皮肤、胃肠道及肝脏症状及实验室检查（1A类）		
	病理诊断		有条件的患者可以穿刺活检，启动治疗不必等待病理结果（1A类）	肝活检诊断aGVHD应权衡风险和获益谨慎采用
分度标准		MAGIC标准、改良Glucksberg标准、IBMTR标准		

【注释】

aGVHD 主要为临床诊断，需要注意排除其他可能情况，尤其在 aGVHD 表现不典型或治疗效果欠佳时，鉴别诊断尤为重要。

1. 皮肤　是 aGVHD 最多累及的靶器官，表现为斑丘疹，多始于头颈部、耳后、面部、肩膀，累及手掌足心较多，无症状或仅有轻度瘙痒或疼痛。需要与预处理毒性、药疹、病毒性皮疹等鉴别诊断（1A 类）。

2. 胃肠道　可以累及上消化道和/或下消化道。上消化道 aGVHD 主要表现厌食、消瘦、恶心呕吐，下消化道 aGVHD 表现为水样腹泻、腹痛、便血和/或肠梗阻。需要与消化性溃疡、感染（如艰难梭菌、CMV、EBV、腺病毒、轮状病毒等）、药物副作用、预处理毒性、血栓性微血管病（TMA）等鉴别诊断（1A 类）。

3. 肝脏　表现为胆汁淤积导致的高胆红素血症，伴有或不伴有肝脏酶谱增高。需要与预处理相关毒性、药物性肝损伤、肝窦阻塞综合征、脓毒症相关性胆汁淤积和病毒性肝炎等鉴别诊断（1A 类）。

目前尚无特异性的生物学标志物达到诊断 aGVHD 的级别，故本指南未推荐[16]。目前主要有三种分度标准，其中临床最常采用改良 Glucksberg 标准，近年研究中 MAGIC 分级系统应用有增多趋势（附录 8~附录 10）。

6.4 急性移植物抗宿主病治疗药物推荐

一线治疗

	I级推荐	II级推荐	III级推荐
治疗启动时机	同胞全合移植和无关供者移植Ⅱ度aGVHD开始启动系统性治疗（1A类）	单倍体移植早期发生的Ⅰ度aGVHD也推荐启动系统性激素治疗（1B类）	治疗启动的时机主要取决于临床症状，推荐治疗前行活检检查，但这不是必需的（2B类）
系统性治疗激素起始剂量	一线治疗是甲泼尼龙1或2mg/（kg·d），或者泼尼松（1A类）		
激素剂量调整原则	如果Ⅰ度aGVHD，或者Ⅱ度aGVHD只累及皮肤或者只累及上消化道，可以应用更低剂量的激素，例如1mg/（kg·d）甲泼尼龙或者泼尼松（1A类）		

一线治疗（续）

	I级推荐	II级推荐	III级推荐
减量更换原则	治激素耐药 GVHD 患者，长期使用激素会引起多种不良反应，推荐启用二线治疗（1A 类）	治疗后达到完全缓解后或者治疗 7 天后激素减量，静脉激素可以改用口服，激素可以用到全部临床症状消失 激素减量推荐慢减，根据治疗反应调整。完全缓解患者，推荐 4 周减至初始剂量的 10%（1B 类）	
其他治疗		口服不吸收的激素，例如布地奈德或口服倍氯米松，可以考虑与系统性激素一起联用治疗胃肠道 aGVHD（1B 类）	同胞全合移植皮肤 I 级 aGVHD 可以考虑局部应用激素，全身应用激素时，也可以考虑局部激素治疗（3 类）*

二线治疗

	Ⅰ级推荐	Ⅱ级推荐	Ⅲ级推荐
启动时机			激素耐药或者激素依赖，可以启动二线治疗（2B类）
治疗方案		目前尚无标准二线治疗。目前倾向于在下列药物中选择：巴利昔单抗、JAK抑制剂（芦可替尼，FDA已经批准）、吗替麦考酚酯、MTX、西罗莫司，间充质干细胞（MSC）治疗，体外光化学治疗，阿仑单抗等	粪菌移植

【注释】

尽管目前aGVHD一线治疗推荐甲泼尼龙剂量为1~2mg/（kg·d），实际临床操作中，各大移植中心在一线激素用量、基础免疫抑制剂应用及激素减量方法上不尽相同。二线治疗方案的最佳选择目前也尚无定论[17]。临床实践中，一线激素用量、基础免疫抑制剂应用及激素减量方法调整需要根据GVHD临床表现、疾病复发、脏器功能及感染等因素统筹考虑。

2017年的一项前瞻随机对照研究证实[18]，新诊断的Ⅰ度aGVHD，接受激素治疗后，与观察组患者相比，感染发生率更高，Ⅲ~Ⅳ度aGVHD的发生率两组类似。故本指南推荐同胞全合及无关供者移植中，新诊断的Ⅰ度aGVHD可以密切观察。应用"北京方案"的单倍体移植系统下[17]，早期发生的Ⅰ度aGVHD也推荐启动系统性激素治疗（1B类）。一项纳入了7项随机对照研究的meta分析证实[17]，aGVHD一线治疗中，加用其他免疫抑制剂（MMF、rATG、英夫利昔单抗、巴利昔单抗等），与单用激素治疗相比，联合治疗组患者的总生存降低14%。更高剂量的激素[如10mg/（kg·d）]，与2mg/（kg·d）甲泼尼龙相比，并不改善生存。*本指南新诊断aGVHD的一线治疗为单用激素。2022年的一项前瞻单臂研究证实，经过临床分度和生物标志物（如基于ST2和REG3α外周血浓度的MAGIC评分等）判定为低危的aGVHD，也可以考虑单用JAK1抑制剂Itacitinib（3类），28天的总反应率可以达到89%，对于激素使用禁忌的aGVHD患者，可以作为治疗的选择[19]。

在Thomas教授编著的《造血干细胞移植》一书中，aGVHD疗效评估时，将一线激素治疗3天评估为进展（PD）、7天评估为无反应（NR）或14天未达CR的情况，定义为激素耐药。在2018年欧洲骨髓移植学会（EBMT）-美国国立综合癌症网络（NCCN）-国际骨髓移植研究中心（NIH-CIBMTR）的标准命名中，aGVHD疗效评估时，将一线激素开始治疗后3~5天内疗效评估为PD或治疗5~7天内疗效评估为NR或包括激素在内的免疫抑制剂治疗28天未达CR的情况定义为激素耐药。此外，将初始一线治疗激素不能减量或激素减量过程中aGVHD再活动定义为激素依赖。激素耐药和激素依赖均为激素治疗失败。目前争议比较大的是aGVHD的二线治疗[20-23]。尚无足够的数据来横向对比各种二线治疗方案的疗效。最近的REACH 2研究比较了芦可替尼与研究者选择的其他二线治疗的疗效[21]：28天CR率，芦可替尼组为62%，明显高于其他治疗组的39%。治疗后6个月失去疗效的比例芦可替尼组10%，其他二线治疗组为39%。抗白细胞介素-2受体抗体（anti-IL-2 receptor antibody，IL-2RA）巴利昔单抗：是国内迄今最多选用的aGVHD二线药物。巴利昔单抗对成人激素耐药aGvHD的总有效率达78.7%~86.8%，CR率达60.9%~69.8%；对儿童HID-HSCT后激素耐药aGVHD的总有效率达85%，CR率74%[22]。

参考文献

[1] XU L, CHEN H, CHEN J, et al. The consensus on indications, conditioning regimen, and donor selection of allogeneic hematopoietic cell transplantation for hematological diseases in China-recommendations from the Chinese Society of Hematology. J Hematol Oncol, 2018, 11 (1): 33.

[2] WANG Y, WU DP, LIU QF, et al. Low-dose post-transplant cyclophosphamide and anti-thymocyte globulin as an effective strategy for GVHD prevention in haploidentical patients. J Hematol Oncol, 2019, 12 (1): 88.

[3] CHANG YJ, WU DP, LAI YR, et al. Antithymocyte globulin for matched sibling donor transplantation in patients with hematologic malignancies: A multicenter, open-label, randomized controlled study. J Clin Oncol, 2020, 38 (29): 3367-3376.

[4] DOU L, HOU C, MA C, et al. Reduced risk of chronic GVHD by low-dose rATG in adult matched sibling donor peripheral blood stem cell transplantation for hematologic malignancies. Ann Hematol, 2020, 99 (1): 167-179.

[5] LI HH, LI F, GAO CJ, et al. Similar incidence of severe acute GVHD and less severe chronic GVHD in PBSCT from unmanipulated, haploidentical donors compared with that from matched sibling donors for patients with haematological malignancies. Br J Haematol, 2017, 176 (1): 92-100.

[6] FINKE J, BETHGE WA, SCHMOOR C, et al. Standard graft-versus-host disease prophylaxis with or without anti-T-cell globulin in haematopoietic cell transplantation from matched unrelated donors: A randomised, open-label, multicentre phase 3 trial. Lancet Oncol, 2009, 10 (9): 855-864.

[7] CHANG YJ, XU LP, WANG Y, et al. Controlled, randomized, open-label trial of risk-stratified corticosteroid prevention of acute graft-versus-host disease after haploidentical transplantation. J Clin Oncol, 2016, 34 (16): 1855-1863.

[8] GAO L, LIU J, ZHANG Y, et al. Low incidence of acute graft-versus-host disease with short-term tacrolimus in haploidentical hematopoietic stem cell transplantation. Leuk Res, 2017, 57: 27-36.

[9] GOOPTU M, KORETH J. Better acute graft-versus-host disease outcomes for allogeneic transplant recipients in the modern era: A tacrolimus effect？. Haematologica, 2017, 102 (5): 806-808.

[10] 朱江, 汤宝林, 宋闯迪, 等. 非血缘脐血干细胞移植与同胞造血干细胞移植治疗 MDS-EB 和 AML-MRC 的对比观察. 中华血液学杂志, 2019, 40 (4): 294-300.

[11] MALARD F, SZYDLO RM, BRISSOT E, et al. Impact of cyclosporine: A concentration on the incidence of severe acute graft-versus-host disease after allogeneic stem cell transplantation. Biol Blood Marrow Transplant, 2010, 16 (1): 28-34.

[12] SCHMID C, SCHLEUNING M, SCHWERDTFEGER R, et al. Long-term survival in refractory acute myeloid leukemia after sequential treatment with chemotherapy and reduced-intensity conditioning for allogeneic stem cell transplantation. Blood, 2006, 108 (3): 1092-1099.

[13] XU LP, JIN S, WANG SQ, et al. Upfront haploidentical transplant for acquired severe aplastic anemia: Registry-based comparison with matched related transplant. J Hematol Oncol, 2017, 10 (1): 25.

[14] KILLICK SB, BOWN N, CAVENAGH J, et al. Guidelines for the diagnosis and management of adult aplastic anaemia. Br J Haematol, 2016, 172 (2): 187-207.

[15] XU LP, JIN S, WANG SQ, et al. Upfront haploidentical transplant for acquired severe aplastic anemia: Registry-

based comparison with matched related transplant. J Hematol Oncol, 2017, 10 (1): 25.
- [16] ALI AM, DIPERSIO JF, SCHROEDER MA. The role of biomarkers in the diagnosis and risk stratification of acute graft-versus-host disease: A systematic review. Biol Blood Marrow Transplant, 2016, 22 (9): 1552-1564.
- [17] 中华医学会血液学分会干细胞应用学组. 中国异基因造血干细胞移植治疗血液系统疾病专家共识 (Ⅲ): 急性移植物抗宿主病 (2020 年版). 中华血液学杂志, 2020, 41 (7): 529-536.
- [18] BACIGALUPO A, MILONE G, CUPRI A, et al. Steroid treatment of acute graft-versus-host disease grade Ⅰ: A randomized trial. Haematologica, 2017, 102 (12): 2125-2133.
- [19] RASHIDI A, DIPERSIO JF, SANDMAIER BM, et al. Steroids versus steroids plus additional agent in frontline treatment of acute graft-versus-host disease: A systematic review and Meta-analysis of randomized trials. Biol Blood Marrow Transplant, 2016, 22 (6): 1133-1137.
- [20] ZEISER R, VON BUBNOFF N, BUTLER J, et al. Ruxolitinib for glucocorticoid-refractory acute graft-versus-host disease. N Engl J Med, 2020, 382 (19): 1800-1810.
- [21] LIU SN, ZHANG XH, XU LP, et al. Prognostic factors and long-term follow-up of basiliximab for steroid-refractory acute graft-versus-host disease: Updated experience from a large-scale study. Am J Hematol, 2020, 95 (8): 927-936.
- [22] TANG FF, CHENG YF, XU LP, et al. Basiliximab as treatment for steroid-refractory acute graft-versus-host disease in pediatric patients after haploidentical hematopoietic stem cell transplantation. Biol Blood Marrow Transplant, 2020, 26 (2): 351-357.

7 异基因造血干细胞移植慢性移植物抗宿主病的预防、诊断及治疗

7.1 慢性移植物抗宿主病的预防

推荐药物	Ⅰ级推荐	Ⅱ级推荐	Ⅲ级推荐
1	钙调磷酸酶抑制剂：CsA（1B类）	钙调磷酸酶抑制剂：FK506（2A类）	
2	ATG 适用于单倍型相合、无关供者造血干细胞移植、40~60 岁亲缘间全相合清髓性 HSCT、亲缘间全相合减低剂量与预处理 HSCT（1A类）		
3	吗替麦考酚酯（MMF）（2A类）		
4	MTX（2A类）		
5	PT/CY（2A类）		
6		MSCs（2A类）	
7		ATG+PT/CY（2B类）	

【注释】

1. 在造血干细胞移植中，对于 GVHD 的预防往往作为一个整体进行统筹，cGVHD 的预防一般是在 aGVHD 预防的基础上，少有专门针对 cGVHD 的预防方案，其发生率也是在现有的 GVHD 预防方案基础上统计而来。移植中不能单单只考虑 cGVHD 发生问题，应充分评估患者的疾病状态、HLA 相合情况等来进行选择[1-2]。

2. 预防 cGVHD 主要依靠药物组合进行，最基本和经典的组合是钙调磷酸酶抑制剂 CsA+ 甲氨蝶呤 MTX（CsA/MTX），有报道 PT/CY 联合短疗程 CsA（5 天开始 CsA 1.5mg/kg，静脉注射，每天两次，250~350µg/L；无 GVHD 患者在第 70 天时停止使用 CSA 而非逐渐减量），有效预防 cGVHD[3]。单倍型相合造血干细胞移植的药物组合比较复杂，"北京方案"采用 ATG+CsA/FK506+MTX+MMF 组合[4]；40~60 岁标危的恶性血液病患者，接受亲缘间全相合移植，使用 ATG 4.5mg/kg，分在 -3~-1 天，联合 CsA、MTX 以及 MMF 能有效降低 GVHD，2 年 cGVHD 发生率为 27.9%，比对照组下降 24.6%[5]。也有尝试亲缘间全相合减低剂量预处理时加入低剂量 ATG（2.5mg/kg，分在 -4~-1 天），有效减低 cGVHD[6]，黄晓军教授团队报道在单倍型相合移植中，"北京方案"ATG 7.5mg/kg 和 10mg/kg 均可有效预防 cGVHD，5 年中重度 cGVHD 发病率为 22.3% 与 17.7%，而 ATG 10mg/kg 可能导致 CMV/EBV 相关死亡率增加，ATG 推荐剂量为 7.5mg/kg[7]。需要强调临床中应该根据疾病状态、移植类型不同和 GVHD 评估风险进行适当增减 ATG 用量；建议儿童基于体重、第一次用药前的绝对淋巴细胞计数和干细胞来源，予个体化的 ATG 治疗（2~10mg/kg），改善移植后 $CD4^+$ 细胞重建并且不增加 GVHD 发生率[8]。

3. 应用 ATG 进行 T 细胞体内去除，同类产品有兔 ATG（rATG）和马 ATG（hATG）[9-10]，国内移植中心也有使用猪 ATG（P-ATG）；也有单位采用西罗莫司（sirolimus）作为 MTX/MMF 的替代用药，常搭配 CsA 或 FK506，一般从移植 -3 天开始用药，持续用药 3~6 个月，维持血药浓度在 5~15ng/ml[11]；也有基于 ATG 基础上的预防方案改良：在 ATG/G-CSF 基础预处理上给予减低剂量 PT/CY（14.5mg/kg，+3、+4 天）有效预防 cGVHD（HR=0.60；P=0.047），GRFS 提高 15%[12]，在氟达拉滨/白消安/阿糖胞苷（FBA）基础上予小剂量 ATG（2.5mg/kg +8 天）和减低剂量 PT/CY（40mg/kg，+3、+4 天）预防 cGVHD，2 年生存率提高 21.3%[13]；在 ATG 基础上联合巴利昔单抗（20mg，0、+4 天），3 年 cGVHD 发病率 12.3%[14]。

4. 药物具体用法：rATG 总用量为 1.5~2.5mg/kg，分在 -5~-2 天使用；hATG 用量 3~5mg/kg，分在 -5~-2 天；pATG，剂量在 25~30mg/kg，分在 -5~-2 天[15]；CsA 1.5~2.5mg/(kg·d) 静脉注射，或者 3~5mg/(kg·d) 口服，药物谷浓度控制在 150~300ng/ml；FK506 0.01~0.05mg/kg 静脉注射或 0.1~0.3mg/(kg·d) 口服，药物谷浓度控制在 5~15ng/ml；MTX 于移植后 +1 天，15mg/m^2，+3、+6 天，10mg/m^2；如果是非血缘 HLA 全相合移植或 HLA 单倍体相合移植，在 +11 天需要增加一剂 MTX（10mg/m^2）；MMF 口服 0.5g/次，2 次/d，1~3 个月。应用 PT/CY 方案预防 GVHD，具体用法：+3、+4 天，静脉注射 CTX 50mg/kg[16]；MSCs：单倍型造血干细胞移植后 +100 天起给予 MSCs 连续输注可有效预防 cGVHD 的发生 [1×10^6/(kg·次)，1 次/月，共 4 次]，有效预防 cGVHD 不增加白血病复发[17]。

5. 在使用常规预防方案他克莫司 ±MTX 或 MMF 的同时，HLA 相合的供者外周血干细胞移植物中去除 naïve T 细胞可有效降低 cGVHD 发生率，接受亲缘全相合和相合无关移植的患者 3 年累计 cGVHD 发病率仅为 7% 和 6%[18]。

7.2 慢性移植物抗宿主病的诊断

	Ⅰ级推荐	Ⅱ级推荐	Ⅲ级推荐
cGVHD 诊断	基于临床表现,至少符合 1 个诊断性征象或至少 1 个高度提示 cGVHD 的区分性征象再联合同一器官或其他器官活检或辅助检查以诊断(1A 类)		

【注释】

1. 慢性移植物抗宿主病(chronicgraft-versus-host disease,cGVHD)传统定义为异基因造血干细胞移植 100 天后出现的移植物抗宿主病,发病率为 30%~70%,是造血干细胞移植的远期重要并发症。

2. cGVHD 临床表现类似自身免疫性疾病,可以累及全身的任何一个或多个器官,临床表现多样,最常累及的是皮肤、口腔、肝脏、泪腺、指甲、胃肠道、生殖道、肌肉关节等。cGVHD 的诊断主要基于临床表现,但应除外其他可能,如感染、药物毒性、第二肿瘤等。诊断性征象,区分性征象详见附录 11[19-20]。

3. cGVHD 诊断明确后需要进行临床评估,以便对患者治疗指征和生存质量、预后进行判定,同时也是疗效评估的重要依据。参照 NIH cGVHD 分级系统根据 8 大受累器官(皮肤、口腔、眼睛、胃肠道、肝脏、肺部、关节/筋膜和生殖道)的严重程度进行划分:0 分指没症状;1 分指没有严重的功能受损，对日常活动没有影响；2 分指对日常活动有明显影响但没残疾；3 分指对日常活动有严重影响伴有严重残疾。cGVHD 的严重程度分级见附录 12。

4. 此外，生物标志物用于 cGVHD 的精准诊断尚不成熟，检测指标包括 T 细胞亚群、细胞因子（cytokine）、趋化因子家族（CXC）、自身抗体（autoantibody）、微小核糖核酸（miRNAs）等，有待进一步研究。但生物标志物在局部器官累积方面有较明确意义，可协助诊断和评估预后，有报道 CXCL9、CCL17 分别在皮肤、肝脏 cGVHD 患者中表达增高[21-23]；IL-8，IFN-γ，CXCL9 及 CCL17 在眼部 cGVHD 患者泪液中表达增高[24]。因此生物标志物在 cGVHD 的诊断模式需要进一步探索。

7.3 慢性移植物抗宿主病的一线治疗

	Ⅰ级推荐	Ⅱ级推荐	Ⅲ级推荐
1	肾上腺皮质激素，如泼尼松（1A类）		
2		泼尼松+CsA/FK506（2B类）	
3		泼尼松+奥法妥木单抗（2B类）	
4		泼尼松+伊布替尼（ibrutinib）（2B类）	

【注释】

1. 治疗原则 应当强调，不是所有cGVHD的患者都需要全身治疗。根据NIH cGVHD的临床评估结果，达到中、重度cGVHD患者需要启动全身治疗，轻度患者仅需要局部治疗或者临床观察。

2. 一线治疗 首选肾上腺皮质激素，联合或不联合钙调磷酸酶抑制剂。如果一线治疗有效，cGVHD症状得到有效控制后，激素逐渐进行减量。激素如何减至今无统一方案，但需把握一个原则：缓慢减量、足够疗程。如果采用的是激素联合CsA等钙调剂治疗，建议首先减激素，其他免疫抑制剂每2~4周减量一次，3~9个月减停一种，免疫抑制剂治疗的中位时间应该足够长，建议整体疗程1~3年[25]。

3. 药物具体用法 泼尼松剂量一般为1mg/（kg·d），单次服用。泼尼松+CsA/FK506；CsA 3~5mg/（kg·d）口服，血药浓度150~200ng/ml或FK506 0.1~0.3mg/（kg·d）口服，0.01~0.05mg/kg静脉注射，每12小时一次，血药浓度5~15ng/ml；奥法妥木单抗的推荐剂量为1 000mg静脉注射，共2次，间隔2周使用，6个月ORR为62.5%[26]。伊布替尼的推荐剂量为420mg口服，1次/d[27]。

7.4 慢性移植物抗宿主病的二线治疗

	Ⅰ级推荐	Ⅱ级推荐	Ⅲ级推荐
1	MTX：每周 1 次，直至 GVHD 症状缓解或副作用不能耐受；如果患者白细胞计数 $<2 \times 10^9/L$，血小板计数 $<50 \times 10^9/L$，用量可减半。欧洲 cGVHD 诊断治疗指南中已将 MTX 列为激素耐药或激素不耐受 cGVHD 的重要的挽救治疗方案（2A 类）		
2	芦可替尼（ruxolitinib）：治疗总体有效率为 85%~100%，CR 在 50% 以上，起效时间比较短；大部分患者能够减少甚至停用激素。如果使用时间长要注意感染发生率高，特别是病毒（如 CMV）再激活的问题（2A 类），其他不良反应主要有血小板减少和贫血		

慢性移植物抗宿主病的二线治疗（续）

	Ⅰ级推荐	Ⅱ级推荐	Ⅲ级推荐
3		伊布替尼（ibrutinib）：总缓解率为67%~79%。与糖皮质激素合用，可显著减少激素用量，延长缓解中位时间（2A类）	
4			利妥昔单抗（rituximab）：可单用；利妥昔单抗联合MMF、FK506或西罗莫司的三联疗法，总缓解率达88%，2年存活率为82%（2B类）
5		伊马替尼（imatinib）：治疗总缓解率在36%~79%，合并肠道、肺部、皮肤病变患者显示出更好的治疗效果（2A类）	

慢性移植物抗宿主病的二线治疗（续）

	I 级推荐	II 级推荐	III 级推荐
6			小剂量 IL-2：有效率为 52%~61%。常见不良反应包括发热、乏力和骨关节疼痛，均为 I~II 级（2B 类）
7	西罗莫司（sirolimus）：可单用，并且与钙调磷酸酶抑制剂类药物具有协同并降低肾毒性的优点，适合 cGVHD 长时间使用（2A 类）		
8		MMF：常与 CsA、MTX 和/或 ATG 联用以预防 GVHD，总缓解率为 69%~72%，不良反应可接受（2A 类）	
9		泊马度胺：具有抗纤维化作用，特别对皮肤和关节受累显示较好治疗效果（2A 类）	

慢性移植物抗宿主病的二线治疗（续）

	I级推荐	II级推荐	III级推荐
10		belumosudil：6个月FFS可达75%，2年的总体生存率可达82%。能够显著降低激素用量，甚至停用激素。对肺部cGVHD症状改善明显（2A类）	
11			axatilimab：总缓解率为67%~82%，对受累器官症状均有缓解作用，常见不良反应包括乏力、恶心、外周性水肿（2B类）

【注释】

1. 启动二线治疗的适应证　①既往累及的器官损伤加重；②出现新的器官受累；③正规用药1个月症状体征没有改善或进展；④泼尼松不能减量到1.0mg/（kg·d）以下或者激素依赖。符合上述指标的可以启动二线治疗[21]。

2. 更换二线治疗药物后需要给予足够的观察期，不要急于短时间换药，一般需观察8~12周，除非4周内病情明显进展才能考虑再次更换其他二线药物[28]。二线治疗目前尚无标准的优选治疗方案，患者可依据个体化状况和靶器官特点尝试选择。

3. 药物具体用法　MTX用量10mg/m^2（静脉注射），在第1、3或4天和第8天重复给药后，每周1次，直至GVHD症状缓解或副作用不能耐受[29]；芦可替尼5~10mg，2次/d，口服[30-31]，或根据体重：5mg，2次/d（体重<60kg），10mg，2次/d（体重>60kg），国内多团队报道芦可替尼5~10mg，2次/d治疗激素耐受cGVHD（SR-cGVHD），ORR为70.7%~74.3%[32-34]。伊布替尼420~560mg口服，直至cGVHD发生进展或毒性无法耐受[35]，儿童伊布替尼治疗cGVHD推荐剂量：<12岁，120mg/m^{2}起始，1次/d，14天后逐渐提升至240mg/m^2；≥12岁，420mg/d，24周ORR为64%[36]。西罗莫司1~2mg/d口服，维持治疗时间3~6个月，有效治疗浓度5~15ng/ml[37]；伊马替尼治疗起始剂量100mg/d，最大量400mg/d，也可直接给药300mg/d，后续调整药量[38]；利妥昔单抗用量375mg/m^2，每周1次，连用4周[39-40]；小剂量IL-2：$1×10^6$IU/m^2，疗程8~12周[41]；吗替麦考酚酯0.5g/次，2次/d[42]；间充质干细胞$1×10^6$/（kg·次），1次/2周，共2~4次，缓解率为57.1%~73.7%[43]。泊马度胺推荐剂量0.5mg/（次·d），口服，6个月ORR达67%[44]；ROCK2抑制剂（belumosudil）200mg，1次/d和200mg，2次/d治疗cGVHD的最佳ORR是74%和77%[45]，也有研究推荐

400mg，1 次/d，肺部 cGVHD 患者 ORR 为 32%[46]；艾克利单抗（axatilimab）用量 1mg/kg，2 周 1 次，7 个治疗周期后 ORR 为 82%[47]。

4. 异基因造血干细胞移植后 cGVHD 发生病理机制复杂，临床表现多样，以造血干细胞移植专科医生为主导，多学科协作的诊治模式有利于 cGVHD 的诊断和治疗。此外，cGVHD 的诊治需和感染（如细菌、真菌、CMV、EB 病毒等感染）相鉴别，感染和排异往往同时存在，相互影响。同时推荐将 cGVHD 作为慢病进行管理，定期随访，逐步提高 cGVHD 患者生活质量，达到治愈目的。

参考文献

[1] ZHANG X, CHEN J, HAN MZ, et al. The consensus from The Chinese Society of Hematology on indications, conditioning regimens and donor selection for allogeneic hematopoietic stem cell transplantation: 2021 update. J Hematol Oncol, 2021, 14: 145.

[2] WANG X, HUANG R, ZHANG X, et al. Current status and prospects of hematopoietic stem cell transplantation in China. Chin Med J (Engl), 2022, 135 (12): 1394-1403.

[3] BROERS A, DE JONG CN, BAKUNINA K, et al. Posttransplant cyclophosphamide for prevention of graft-versus-host disease: Results of the prospective randomized HOVON-96 trial. Blood Adv, 2022, 6 (11): 3378-3385.

[4] HUANG XJ, LIU DH, LIU KY, et al. Haploidentical hematopoietic stem cell transplantation without in vitro T-cell depletion for the treatment of hematological malignancies. Bone Marrow Transplant, 2006, 38 (4): 291-297.

[5] CHANG YJ, WU DP, LAI YR, et al. Antithymocyte globulin for matched sibling donor transplantation in patients with hematologic malignancies: A multicenter, open-label, randomized controlled study. J Clin Oncol, 2020, 38 (29): 3367-

3376.

[6] MOHTY M, BAY JO, FAUCHER C, et al. Graft-versus-host disease following allogeneic transplantation from HLA-identical sibling with antithymocyte globulin-based reduced-intensity preparative regimen. Blood, 2003, 102 (2): 470-476.

[7] WANG Y, LIU QF, LIN R, et al. Optimizing antithymocyte globulin dosing in haploidentical hematopoietic cell transplantation: Long-term follow-up of a multicenter, randomized controlled trial. Sci Bull (Beijing), 2021, 66 (24): 2498-2505.

[8] ADMIRAAL R, NIERKENS S, BIERINGS MB, et al. Individualised dosing of anti-thymocyte globulin in paediatric unrelated allogeneic haematopoietic stem-cell transplantation (PARACHUTE): A single-arm, phase 2 clinical trial. Lancet Haematol, 2022, 9 (2): e111-e120.

[9] LUO Y, JIN M, TAN Y, et al. Antithymocyte globulin improves GVHD-free and relapse-free survival in unrelated hematopoietic stem cell transplantation. Bone Marrow Transplant, 2019, 54 (10): 1668-1675.

[10] CHEN X, WEI J, HUANG Y, et al. Effect of Antithymocyte globulin source on outcomes of hla-matched sibling allogeneic hematopoietic stem cell transplantation for patients with severe aplastic anemia. Biol Blood Marrow Transplant, 2018, 24 (1): 86-90.

[11] FENG Y, CHEN X, CASSADY K, et al. The role of mTOR inhibitors in hematologic disease: From bench to bedside. Front Oncol, 2020, 10: 611690.

[12] WANG Y, WU DP, LIU QF, et al. Low-dose post-transplant cyclophosphamide and anti-thymocyte globulin as an effective strategy for GVHD prevention in haploidentical patients. J Hematol Oncol, 2019, 12 (1): 88.

[13] ZHANG W, GUI R, ZU Y, et al. Reduced-dose post-transplant cyclophosphamide plus low-dose post-transplant anti-thymocyte globulin as graft-versus-host disease prophylaxis with fludarabine-busulfan-cytarabine conditioning in haploidentical peripheral blood stem cell transplantation: A multicentre, randomized controlled clinical trial. Br J

Haematol, 2023, 200 (2): 210-221.

[14] HUANG Z, YAN H, TENG Y, et al. Lower dose of ATG combined with basiliximab for haploidentical hematopoietic stem cell transplantation is associated with effective control of GVHD and less CMV viremia. Front Immunol, 2022, 13: 1017850.

[15] GORIN NC. How antithymocyte globulin, a polyclonal soup of the past century, when carefully dosed, has become crucial for hematopoietic stem cell transplantation with haplo-identical donors in the 21st century. Sci Bull (Beijing), 2021, 66 (24): 2445-2447.

[16] BRISSOT E, LABOPIN M, MOISEEV I, et al. Post-transplant cyclophosphamide versus antithymocyte globulin in patients with acute myeloid leukemia in first complete remission undergoing allogeneic stem cell transplantation from 10/10 HLA-matched unrelated donors. J Hematol Oncol, 2020, 13 (1): 87.

[17] GAO L, ZHANG Y, HU B, et al. Phase Ⅱ multicenter, randomized, double-blind controlled study of efficacy and safety of umbilical cord-derived mesenchymal stromal cells in the prophylaxis of chronic graft-versus-host disease after HLA-haploidentical stem-cell transplantation. J Clin Oncol, 2016, 34 (24): 2843-2850.

[18] BLEAKLEY M, SEHGAL A, SEROPIAN S, et al. Naive T-cell depletion to prevent chronic graft-versus-host disease. J Clin Oncol, 2022, 40 (11): 1174-1185.

[19] KITKO CL, PIDALA J, SCHOEMANS HM, et al. National institutes of health consensus development project on criteria for clinical trials in chronic graft-versus-host disease: IIa. The 2020 Clinical Implementation and Early Diagnosis Working Group Report. Transplant Cell Ther, 2021, 27 (7): 545-557.

[20] BUXBAUM NP, SOCIÉ G, HILL GR, et al. Chronic GvHD NIH Consensus Project Biology Task Force: Evolving path to personalized treatment of chronic GvHD. Blood Adv, 2022: 2022007611.

[21] 中华医学会血液学分会造血干细胞应用学组, 中国抗癌协会血液病转化委员会. 慢性移植物抗宿主病 (cGVHD) 诊断与治疗中国专家共识 (2021 年版). 中华血液学杂志, 2021, 42 (4): 265-275.

[22] WANG W, HONG T, WANG X, et al. Newly found peacekeeper: potential of CD8+ Tregs for Graft-Versus-Host Disease. Front Immunol, 2021, 12: 764786.

[23] LI X, CHEN T, GAO Q, et al. A panel of 4 biomarkers for the early diagnosis and therapeutic efficacy of aGVHD. JCI Insight, 2019, 4 (16): 130413.

[24] CHENG X, HUANG R, HUANG S, et al. Recent advances in ocular graft-versus-host disease. Front Immunol, 2023, 14: 1092108.

[25] FLOWERS ME, MARTIN PJ. How we treat chronic graft-versus-host disease. Blood, 2015, 125 (4): 606-615.

[26] LAZARYAN A, LEE S, ARORA M, et al. A phase 2 multicenter trial of ofatumumab and prednisone as initial therapy for chronic graft-versus-host disease. Blood Adv, 2022, 6 (1): 259-269.

[27] MIKLOS DB, ABU ZAID M, COONEY JP, et al. Ibrutinib for first-line treatment of chronic graft-versus-host disease: Results from the randomized phase Ⅲ iNTEGRATE study. J Clin Oncol, 2023: JCO2200509.

[28] 冯一梅, 张曦. 重视慢性移植物抗宿主病的临床管理. 临床血液学杂志, 2019, 32 (9): 651-655.

[29] WANG Y, XU LP, LIU DH, et al. First-line therapy for chronic graft-versus-host disease that includes low-dose methotrexate is associated with a high response rate. Biol Blood Marrow Transplant, 2009, 15 (4): 505-511.

[30] ZHAO JY, LIU SN, XU LP, et al. Ruxolitinib is an effective salvage treatment for multidrug-resistant graft-versus-host disease after haploidentical allogeneic hematopoietic stem cell transplantation without posttransplant cyclophosphamide. Ann Hematol, 2021, 100 (1): 169-180.

[31] ZEISER R, POLVERELLI N, RAM R, et al. Ruxolitinib for glucocorticoid-refractory chronic graft-versus-host disease. N Engl J Med, 2021, 385 (3): 228-238.

[32] WU H, SHI J, LUO Y, et al. Evaluation of ruxolitinib for steroid-refractory chronic graft-vs-host disease after allogeneic hematopoietic stem cell transplantation. JAMA Netw Open, 2021, 4 (1): e2034750.

[33] WANG D, LIU Y, LAI X, et al. Efficiency and Toxicity of ruxolitinib as a salvage treatment for steroid-refractory

chronic graft-versus-host disease. Front Immunol, 2021, 12: 673636.
[34] FAN S, HUO WX, YANG Y, et al. Efficacy and safety of ruxolitinib in steroid-refractory graft-versus-host disease: A meta-analysis. Front Immunol, 2022, 13: 954268.
[35] MIKLOS D, CUTLER CS, ARORA M, et al. Ibrutinib for chronic graft-versus-host disease after failure of prior therapy. Blood, 2017, 130 (21): 2243-2250.
[36] CARPENTER PA, KANG HJ, YOO KH, et al. Ibrutinib treatment of pediatric chronic graft-versus-host disease: Primary results from the phase 1/2 iMAGINE study. Transplant Cell Ther, 2022, 28 (11): 771e1-771e10.
[37] 朱雯, 冯一梅, 陈婷, 等. 西罗莫司联合钙调磷酸酶抑制剂治疗糖皮质激素耐药/依赖广泛型慢性移植物抗宿主病临床观察. 中华血液学杂志, 2020, 41 (9): 716-722.
[38] BAIRD K, COMIS LE, JOE GO, et al. Imatinib mesylate for the treatment of steroid-refractory sclerotic-type cutaneous chronic graft-versus-host disease. Biol Blood Marrow Transplant, 2015, 21 (6): 1083-1090.
[39] SOLOMON SR, SIZEMORE CA, RIDGEWAY M, et al. Corticosteroid-free primary treatment of chronic extensive graft-versus-host disease incorporating rituximab. Biol Blood Marrow Transplant, 2015, 21 (9): 1576-1582.
[40] LI X, GAO Q, FENG Y, et al. Developing role of B cells in the pathogenesis and treatment of chronic GVHD. Br J Haematol, 2019, 184 (3): 323-336.
[41] KORETH J, KIM HT, JONES KT, et al. Efficacy, durability, and response predictors of low-dose interleukin-2 therapy for chronic graft-versus-host disease. Blood, 2016, 128 (1): 130-137.
[42] BUSCA A, LOCATELLI F, MARMONT F, et al. Response to mycophenolate mofetil therapy in refractory chronic graft-versus-host disease. Haematologica, 2003, 88 (7): 837-839.
[43] HERRMANN R, STURM M, SHAW K, et al. Mesenchymal stromal cell therapy for steroid-refractory acute and chronic graft versus host disease: A phase 1 study. Int J Hematol, 2012, 95 (2): 182-188.
[44] CURTIS LM, OSTOJIC A, VENZON DJ, et al. A randomized phase 2 trial of pomalidomide in subjects failing prior

therapy for chronic graft-versus-host disease. Blood, 2021, 137 (7): 896-907.

[45] CUTLER C, LEE SJ, ARAI S, et al. Belumosudil for chronic graft-versus-host disease after 2 or more prior lines of therapy: The ROCKstar Study. Blood, 2021, 138 (22): 2278-2289.

[46] DEFILIPP Z, KIM HT, YANG Z, et al. Clinical response to belumosudil in bronchiolitis obliterans syndrome: A combined analysis from 2 prospective trials. Blood Adv, 2022, 6 (24): 6263-6270.

[47] KITKO CL, ARORA M, DEFILIPP Z, et al. Axatilimab for chronic graft-versus-host disease after failure of at least two prior systemic therapies: Results of a phase Ⅰ/Ⅱ study. J Clin Oncol, 2022: JCO2200958.

8 异基因造血干细胞移植过程中真菌感染的预防及治疗

8.1 真菌感染的预防

	I 级推荐	II 级推荐	III 级推荐
适用人群	所有接受异基因移植的患者		
预防药物 [a]	泊沙康唑（1A 类）[1] 米卡芬净（1A 类）[2] 氟康唑 [b][3] 伏立康唑（1A 类）[4] 卡泊芬净（2A 类）[5] 既往确诊或临床诊断侵袭性真菌病（IFD）患者，首选既往抗真菌治疗有效药物		
预防疗程	从接受预处理开始，无/轻度 GVHD 患者一般至少用至移植后 3 个月，有 ≥ II aGVHD 或 ≥ 中重度 cGVHD 患者疗程应延长至 GVHD 临床症状控制，免疫抑制剂基本减停为止		

注：a. 用药推荐不分先后顺序；b. 仅推荐应用于霉菌感染低危患者，如同胞相合移植，患者既往无曲霉菌感染等情况。

【注释】

研究提示当 IFD 发生率 ≥ 5% 人群可通过抗真菌预防治疗获益，IFD 发生率 ≥ 10% 的高危人群获益更显著[6]。我国异基因造血干细胞移植中 HLA 全相合亲缘供体、HLA 相合非血缘供体和亲缘半相合供体移植组确诊和临床诊断 IFD 累计发生率分别达到 4.3%、13.2% 和 12.8%[7]，合并 GVHD，需要接受长期、强免疫抑制治疗的患者是 IFD 发生的高危因素[8]。因此绝大多数异基因造血干细胞移植患者可以从真菌预防治疗中获益。但在接受药物预防之外，患者还应受到全方位的保护措施，包括入住层流病房，远离施工场地、绿植和鲜花等，以减少真菌暴露机会。预防抗真菌药物的选择全球没有统一标准，原则是抗菌谱广、疗效明确且副作用少。具体药物的选择需要结合各单位真菌感染谱、患者各脏器功能、既往用药情况以及药物间作用等综合评估。预防的具体时间取决于患者免疫状态的恢复情况，一般至少移植后 3 个月。

8.2 真菌感染的治疗

	I 级推荐	II 级推荐	III 级推荐
适用人群	**经验治疗**：持续粒缺或者免疫低下人群（IFD 高危患者）发热且经广谱抗细菌药物治疗 4~7 天无效 **诊断驱动治疗**：IFD 低危患者出现影像学异常或者血清 GM/G 试验阳性等相关微生物学 IFD 诊断依据时 **目标治疗**：临床诊断和确诊 IFD 患者		
治疗药物	**经验治疗** [a]： 卡泊芬净（1A 类）[9] 脂质体两性霉素 B（1B 类）[10] 两性霉素 B（1B 类）[11] 米卡芬净（2B 类）[12] 伏立康唑（1B 类）[13] **诊断驱动治疗** [a]： 药物同经验治疗 **目标治疗**： 依据真菌种类、药物抗菌谱、药敏结果、患者具体情况选择用药 [b]		已应用广谱抗真菌药物的患者经验或者诊断驱动治疗时，建议更换为另一种类型抗真菌药物 有条件的单位建议进行伏立康唑、泊沙康唑血药浓度的检测（3 类）[14] 对于单药治疗失败或无法耐受、多部位或耐药真菌感染的高危病例，可采用两种药物进行联合治疗，一般为多烯类或唑类药物与棘白菌素联合（2B 类）[15] 对于确诊病例，建议进行菌种鉴定和药敏检测，根据菌种和药敏进行针对性治疗及管理

真菌感染的治疗(续)

	I 级推荐	II 级推荐	III 级推荐
治疗疗程	对于经验性治疗和诊断驱动治疗患者来说,应用至体温降至正常、临床状况稳定、各项指标好转以及免疫抑制状态改善 诊断驱动治疗还应包括 IFD 相关微生物学和/或影像学指标恢复正常 目标治疗根据感染部位、真菌种类和患者情况而定 [b]		
疗效评估	需结合临床症状、体征、影像学和微生物学结果综合评估 影像学评估:临床症状和体征明显好转患者推荐治疗 14 天后复查 CT G/GM 不推荐作为疗效评估尤其是抗真菌治疗停药的唯一指标		

注:a. 用药推荐不分先后顺序。

b. 念珠菌血症:卡泊芬净和米卡芬净为初始推荐药物,其余可备选药物为氟康唑、两性霉素 B、脂质体两性霉素 B、伏立康唑。治疗应持续至临床症状和体征恢复,且确认血流病原学清除后 2 周以上。

播散性念珠菌病：临床情况稳定，无中性粒细胞缺乏者可首选用氟康唑治疗；伴中性粒细胞缺乏、治疗无效或临床情况不稳定患者，选用棘白菌素类、两性霉素 B 及其脂质体和伏立康唑。治疗持续至血培养转阴和影像学提示病灶完全吸收，常需数月。

中枢神经系统念珠菌病：两性霉素脂质体或联合氟胞嘧啶及伏立康唑为推荐药物。氟康唑可作为临床症状稳定，无粒细胞缺乏且体外药敏敏感患者的治疗。治疗持续至临床症状、体征和影像学异常完全恢复后至少 4 周。

侵袭性曲霉菌病：推荐应用伏立康唑。脂质体两性霉素 B、卡泊芬净和米卡芬净作为备选药物。根据临床严重程度、相关症状和体征恢复速度以及免疫抑制状态改善决定治疗疗程，一般 6~12 周，甚至更长时间。

中枢神经系统曲霉菌病：伏立康唑首选，脂质体两性霉素 B 备选。

毛霉菌病：脂质体两性霉素或两性霉素 B 为首选治疗；泊沙康唑或泊沙康唑联合两性霉素 B 可作为备选方案。除药物治疗外，往往需要联合外科干预或者控制患者基础疾病。

【注释】

经验治疗以持续粒细胞缺乏伴发热且广谱抗菌药物治疗无效作为启动治疗的主要标准，推荐适用于 IFD 高危患者或无条件进行 GM/G 检测的情况下，开始治疗的时间早晚与发生患者 IFD 风险大小相关，通常在发热 4 天或更长时间后开始。血液病患者 IFD 病原体中曲霉菌多见，因此经验性抗菌治疗药物一般选择覆盖曲霉菌的广谱抗真菌药物。与经验治疗比较，诊断驱动治疗不以发热为启动治疗指标，更适合于 IFD 低危患者。无论是经验治疗还是诊断驱动治疗，都应尽可能寻找完善真菌感染证据,除高分辨肺CT、GM/G试验外,支气管镜肺泡灌洗液检查,肺穿刺活检,中枢、腹部等其他部位影像学检查,以及真菌PCR或者宏基因组测序等都是可采用的技术手段。开始治疗后,需要密切评估患者临床表现和影像以及实验室指标,不断修正诊断调整治疗。可选择的药物需要临床医生根据各单位的流行病学、患者不同治疗时期不同真菌感染的概率来综合评估。IFD目标治疗由于感染病原菌较为明确,可依据真菌种类、药物抗菌谱、患者具体情况选择用药。

为对真菌的治疗更加有针对性,对来自血和其他无菌部位(如脑脊液、胸腔积液、脑脓肿等)分离出的真菌、需要长期抗真菌治疗或抗真菌治疗效果不佳时建议进行体外药敏试验,以更好地指导临床应用药物。必须指出的是,真菌药敏试验采用"90/60规则",这意味着由敏感菌株引起的感染中,90%的概率治疗有效,而由耐药菌株引起的感染60%病例也可能治疗成功。

在预防或治疗失败或者怀疑有药物相关副作用时可以进行伏立康唑、泊沙康唑的治疗性药物浓度监测(TDM)明确是否存在药物浓度不足或药物过量。

宿主中性粒细胞数量和功能异常以及免疫抑制状态是IFD危险因素,而中性粒细胞和免疫功能恢复则与IFD治疗预后相关。临床适当减停免疫抑制剂,粒细胞集落刺激因子应用和/或中性粒细胞输注有助于IFD治疗。此外,出现①急性咯血;②为获得组织学诊断;③预防已有累及血管的真菌病灶出血;④去除残留病灶;⑤曲霉菌感染性鼻窦炎、感染性心内膜炎、骨髓炎和关节炎等情况可考虑手术干预。

参考文献

[1] ULLMANN AJ, LIPTON JH, VESOLE DH, et al. Posaconazole or fluconazole forprophylaxis in severe graft-versus-host disease. N Engl J Med, 2007, 356 (4): 335-347.

[2] VAN BURIK JA, RATANATHARATHORN V, STEPAN DE, et al. Micafungin versus fluconazole for prophylaxis against invasive fungal infections during neutropenia in patients undergoing hematopoietic stem cell transplantation. Clin Infect Dis, 2004, 39 (10): 1407-1416.

[3] MARR KA, SEIDEL K, SLAVIN MA, et al. Prolonged fluconazole prophylaxis is associated with persistent protection against candidiasis-related death in allogeneic marrow transplant recipients: Long-term follow-up of a randomized, placebo-controlled trial. Blood, 2000, 96 (6): 2055-2061.

[4] MARKS DI, PAGLIUCA A, KIBBLER CC, et al. Voriconazole versus itraconazole forantifungal prophylaxis following allogeneic haematopoietic stem-cell transplantation. Br J Haematol, 2011, 155 (3): 318-327.

[5] CHOU LS, LEWIS RE, IPPOLITI C, et al. Caspofungin as primary antifungal prophylaxis in stem cell transplantrecipients. Pharmacotherapy, 2007, 27 (12): 1644-1650.

[6] ROGERS TR, SLAVIN MA, DONNELLY JP. Antifungal prophylaxis during treatment for haematological malignancies: Are we there yet ?. Br J Haematol, 2011, 153 (6): 681-697.

[7] SUN Y, MENG FY, HAN MZ, et al. Epidemiology, management, and outcome of invasive fungal disease in patients undergoing hematopoietic stem cell transplantation in China: A multicenter prospective observational study. Biol Blood Marrow Transplant, 2015, 21 (6): 1117-1126.

[8] DOUGLAS AP, SLAVIN MA. Risk factors and prophylaxis against invasive fungal disease for haematology and stem

cell transplant recipients: An evolving field. Expert Rev Anti Infect Ther, 2016, 14 (12): 1165-1177.

[9] WALSH TJ, TEPPLER H, DONOWITZ GR, et al. Caspofungin versus liposomal amphotericin B for empirical antifungal therapy in patients with persistent fever and neutropenia. N Engl J Med, 2004, 351 (14): 1391-1402.

[10] WALSH TJ, FINBERG RW, ARNDT C, et al. Liposomal amphotericin B for empirical therapy in patients with persistent fever and neutropenia: National Institute of Allergy and Infectious Diseases Mycoses Study Group. N Engl J Med, 1999, 340 (10): 764-771.

[11] WINSTON DJ, HATHORN JW, SCHUSTER MG, et al. A multicenter randomized trial of fluconazole versus amphotericin B for empiric antifungal therapy of febrile neutropenic patients with cancer. Am J Med, 2000, 108 (4): 282-289.

[12] OYAKE T, KOWATA S, MURAI K, et al. Comparison of micafungin and voriconazole as empirical antifungal therapies in febrile neutropenic patients with hematological disorders: A randomized controlled trial. Eur J Haematol, 2016, 96 (6): 602-609.

[13] WALSH TJ, PAPPAS P, WINSTON DJ, et al. Voriconazole compared with liposomal amphotericin B for empirical antifungal therapy in patients with neutropenia and persistent fever. N Engl J Med, 2002, 346 (4): 225-234.

[14] TISSOT F, AGRAWAL S, PAGANO L, et al. ECIL-6 guidelines for the treatment of invasive candidiasis, aspergillosis and mucormycosis in leukemia and hematopoietic stem cell transplant patients. Haematologica, 2017, 102 (3): 433-444.

[15] CANDONI A, CAIRA M, CESARO S, et al. Multicentre surveillance study on feasibility, safety and efficacy of antifungal combination therapy for proven or probable invasive fungal diseases in haematological patients: The SEIFEM real-life combo study. Mycoses, 2014, 57 (6): 342-350.

9 异基因造血干细胞移植过程中病毒感染的检测、预防及治疗

9.1 异基因造血干细胞移植中乙型病毒性肝炎管理

9.1.1 HSCT后乙型肝炎病毒（HBV）再激活/感染及疾病的监测[1-4]

	I级推荐	II级推荐	III级推荐
移植前检查	供受者检测HBsAg、抗-HBc和抗-HBs HBsAg阳性或抗-HBc阳性时检测HBV-DNA（1A类）		
HBV再激活/感染风险评估	高风险患者定义为具有以下条件之一者：HBsAg+或抗-HBc+患者 HBV-患者接受HBsAg阳性或抗-HBc阳性移植物或血制品（1A类）		
移植后HBV监测	HBV再激活高风险患者如未接受药物治疗，应密切监测有无HBV再激活 接受药物治疗者，在治疗期间定期监测；停药后仍需定期监测有无HBV再激活（2A类）		

注：HBV，乙型肝炎病毒；HBsAg，乙肝表面抗原；抗-HBc，乙肝核心抗体；抗-HBs，乙肝表面抗体。

9.1.2 HBV 感染患者的 HSCT 时机[1]

	Ⅰ级推荐	Ⅱ级推荐	Ⅲ级推荐
移植时机	HBsAg 阳性或抗-HBc 阳性，且 HBV-DNA 阴性患者 HSCT 前给予抗 HBV 药物治疗，按期移植 活动性 HBV 感染（活检证实慢性肝炎活动，或 HBsAg 阳性且 HBV-DNA 高水平 [a] 患者应尽可能推迟 HSCT，并予药物治疗。然而，HBV-DNA 阳性并非移植的绝对禁忌证（2A 类）		

注：a. 活动性 HBV 感染患者 HBV-DNA 高水平，通常是指 HBV-DNA$>2 \times 10^7$IU/ml [4-5]。

9.1.3 HSCT 患者 HBV 再激活/感染的防治 [1-4]

	Ⅰ级推荐	Ⅱ级推荐	Ⅲ级推荐
抗病毒药物治疗适应证	HBsAg 阳性或抗-HBc 阳性患者 [a]（1A 类）		接受 HBsAg 阳性或抗-HBc 阳性移植物或血制品的 HBV-患者（3 类）
抗病毒药物选择	首选第三代抗 HBV 药物（恩替卡韦、替诺福韦）次选第一代抗 HBV 药物（拉米夫定）（1A 类）		
抗病毒药物治疗疗程 [b]			HBsAg 阳性患者：HSCT 前 1 周开始，持续至少 12 个月 抗-HBc 阳性且 HBsAg 阴性患者：HSCT 前 1 周开始，持续至少 18 个月（3 类）
HBV 疫苗接种 [c]			

【注释】

a 国外指南对于抗-HBc 阳性且 HBsAg 阴性患者（既往感染），推荐药物预防 HBV 再激活或 HSCT 后 12 个月内坚持规律的随访，即每 3 个月监测 HBsAg 和 HBV-DNA。如果 HBV-DNA<1 000IU/ml，每月监测 1 次；出现 HBsAg 阳性或 HBV-DNA>1 000IU/ml 时立即予药物治疗[3]。然而，国内多数中心对既往感染者进行定期随访，未进行常规药物预防 HBV 再激活，鼓励有条件的单位做相关的临床研究。

b 对于药物治疗最佳持续时间仍存在争议[2]。尽管如此，对于 HBsAg 阳性患者推荐药物治疗至少在 HSCT 前 1 周开始，并持续至少 12 个月。如果 HBV-DNA 和 HBsAg 转阴的同时出现抗-HBs 阳性，表明病毒已被清除，抗病毒治疗可停止。对于既往感染者，推荐药物治疗持续至少 18 个月。患者如合并慢性 GVHD 或持续应用免疫抑制剂建议延长抗 HBV 治疗时间。对于接受 HBsAg 阳性或抗-HBc 阳性移植物或血制品的 HBV 阴性患者，药物治疗的维持时间尚不明确。

c 国外指南[2, 6]建议接受 HSCT 的 HBV 阴性患者在预处理前均应接受 HBV 疫苗接种，并定期监测其抗 HBs 效价（Ⅰ级推荐）。移植前 HBV 阴性患者如未在移植前接种疫苗应在移植+6 个月后接受 HBV 疫苗接种（Ⅰ级推荐）。移植前抗-HBc 阳性患者定期评估抗-HBs 抗体效价；若无保护效价应接种疫苗。HBsAg 阴性且抗-HBc 阳性供者在捐献前接种疫苗（Ⅱ级推荐）。HBV 阴性供者 HSCT 前接种疫苗（Ⅲ级推荐）。目前国内多数单位对移植供受者没有常规给予疫苗接种，鼓励进行相关的临床研究[7]。

造血干细胞移植后 HBV 感染/再激活的定义见附录 13；乙肝血清免疫学标志物检测内容及意义见附录 14。

9.2 造血干细胞移植中巨细胞病毒感染管理

9.2.1 HSCT 中巨细胞病毒（CMV）感染/激活及疾病的监测[8-12]

	Ⅰ级推荐	Ⅱ级推荐	Ⅲ级推荐
移植前 CMV 监测	移植前检测供受者外周血 CMV-IgG 抗体（2A 类）		移植前检测供受者外周血 CMV-DNA（3 类）
受者选择	CMV 血清学阴性患者应尽可能选择血清学阴性供者（1A 类）		CMV 血清学阳性患者，应选择 CMV 血清学阳性供者（2B 类）血清学阳性或阴性的供者均适合作为供者（2B 类）
移植后 CMV 监测 a	allo-HSCT 后定期监测患者外周血 CMV-DNA（2A 类）		

【注释】

a 外周血 CMV-DNA 监测推荐定量 PCR（qPCR）检测 CMV-DNA，标本可采用全血、血浆、血清，何种标本最佳尚无定论[9]；传统的 CMV 抗原（pp65）作为 CMV 监测现不推荐。CMV 阳性阈值目前尚无国际公认标准，需结合本单位情况制订[8]。多种指南均推荐在移植后至少 100 天内每周检测 1 次外周血 CMV-DNA，高危（移植前患者血清学阳性、替代供者移植、急性及慢性 GVHD、长期使用糖皮质激素、T 细胞重建延迟等）患者需延长监测时间到 6~12 个月[8, 10-11, 13]。CMV 感染 / 再激活的诊断见附录 15，危险因素见附录 16。

9.2.2 CMV 感染 / 激活的预防治疗 a [14-19]

	I 级推荐	II 级推荐	III 级推荐
原发性 CMV 感染 / 激活的预防		对于 CMV IgG 阴性患者，为避免发生输血传播的原发性 CMV 感染，建议输注 CMV 血清学阴性或去白细胞血制品（2A 类）	
预防指征	高危患者（单倍型移植、脐血造血干细胞移植、接受 ATG 预处理等）		
预防治疗	来特莫韦（1A 类）		
预防治疗的时机	移植后 28 天内启动，持续至移植后 100 天（1A 类）		

【注释】

a 近期发表的随机对照研究显示,移植后 28~100 天使用来特莫韦进行预防能有效减少 CMV 激活,因此来特莫韦也获得国际指南的推荐[15-16]。EBMT 的问卷调查显示:欧洲约有 62% 的移植中心将来特莫韦用于高危患者(单倍型移植、脐血造血干细胞移植、接受 ATG 预处理等)的 CMV 激活预防[17];对于高危人群,特别是急慢性 GVHD 患者,可考虑适当延长疗程或重新启动 CMV 激活预防,应用至免疫抑制剂减量[18-19]。来特莫韦在中国上市以来,越来越多的中心将来特莫韦用于高危人群的 CMV 感染/激活的预防治疗。

9.2.3 CMV 感染/激活的抢先治疗 a [8, 10-12, 21]

	Ⅰ级推荐	Ⅱ级推荐	Ⅲ级推荐
治疗指征	CMV-DNA 血症(1A 类)		抢先治疗的 CMV-DNA 阳性阈值应根据各单位所采用的检测技术和移植体系调整(2B 类)
一线抢先治疗	静脉注射更昔洛韦或膦甲酸钠(1A 类)	缬更昔洛韦,严重胃肠道 GVHD 患者除外(2A 类)	CMV-CTL 联合抗病毒药物(3 类)

CMV 感染/激活的抢先治疗（续）

	Ⅰ级推荐	Ⅱ级推荐	Ⅲ级推荐
二线抢先治疗			西多福韦（2B类） 联合使用半量的膦甲酸钠与半量的更昔洛韦（2B类） CMV-CTL、来氟米特、青蒿琥酯、脂质体西多福韦、maribavir（3类） 酌情减量免疫抑制剂（3类）

注：CMV-CTL.巨细胞病毒特异性细胞毒性T细胞。

【注释】

a 预防即针对CMV血症给予抢先治疗[8,10-11]。目前无统一的启动抢先治疗的CMV-DNA阳性阈值。更昔洛韦和膦甲酸钠作为一线药物选择[22]，更昔洛韦因其骨髓抑制作用，建议白细胞计数$<0.5 \times 10^9$/L或血小板计数$<20 \times 10^9$/L的患者谨慎使用；膦甲酸钠的主要不良反应为肾毒性[22]。抢先治疗疗程至少2周，直至CMV转阴。抢先治疗前2周内CMV-DNA载量升高，无须更改药物。如果治疗2周后CMV仍不转阴，可考虑每天给予一次抗病毒治疗的维持治疗[8]。

9.2.4 CMV 疾病的治疗 a [8, 10-11, 23]

	Ⅰ级推荐	Ⅱ级推荐	Ⅲ级推荐
治疗药物	更昔洛韦（2A 类） 膦甲酸钠（2A 类）		西多福韦（2B 类） 联用全量的膦甲酸钠与全量的更昔洛韦（2B 类） 玻璃体内注射更昔洛韦或膦甲酸钠治疗 CMV 视网膜炎（2B 类） 缬更昔洛韦（重度胃肠道 GVHD 除外）（3 类）
IVIG 或高效价 CMV 特异性丙种球蛋白			CMV 肺炎患者推荐使用 IVIG 或高效价 CMV 特异性丙种球蛋白（3 类）
免疫抑制剂调整			酌情减量免疫抑制剂（3 类）
CMV 过继免疫治疗			allo-HSCT 后难治性 CMV 感染可使用 CML-CTL 治疗（2B 类）

【注释】

a CMV 疾病的治疗分为诱导和维持治疗，疗程尚无定论。诱导治疗是指开始治疗至症状缓解且外周血 CMV 转阴，通常需要 3~4 周；当 CMV 转阴后继续维持治疗 2~4 周[10]。CMV 疾病的一线与二线抗病毒药物选择与抢先治疗相同[8, 11]。更昔洛韦联合膦甲酸钠并不能增加疗效，但往往会增加毒性。西多福韦联合更昔洛韦或膦甲酸钠可能提高疗效[23-26]。CMV 耐药较少见，若治疗 2 周后 CMV 定量增加、伴或不伴 CMV 疾病临床表现的进展，则考虑存在 CMV 耐药，需更换为二线治疗[8]。

CMV 感染治疗的常用药及用法见附录 17。

9.2.5 CMV 耐药 a[8]

	I 级推荐	II 级推荐	III 级推荐
耐药检测			临床怀疑 CMV 耐药时，应进行 CMV 耐药检测（3 类）
治疗		马立巴韦（2A 类）b	
药物调整		耐药检测结果回报前，应对病毒载量上升或疾病恶化的患者进行治疗调整（2B 类）	

【注释】

a CMV 耐药机制包括基因突变所致的耐药和缺少基因突变的临床耐药[24]。CMV 耐药定义：①难治性 CMV 感染，外周血病毒载量经至少 2 周的适当抗病毒治疗后增加超过 1 个对数级；②临床诊断难治性 CMV 感染，外周血病毒载量经至少 2 周的适当抗病毒治疗后维持原来水平或升高不超过 1 个对数级；③难治性 CMV 终末器官疾病，经至少 2 周的适当抗病毒治疗后临床症状或体征恶化，或进展为终末器官疾病[25-26]；④临床诊断难治性 CMV 终末器官疾病，经至少 2 周的适当抗病毒治疗后临床症状或体征无改善；⑤抗病毒药物耐药，一个或多个基因突变所致的耐药。

b 最新的一项马立巴韦治疗难治性 CMV 感染的 3 期 RCT 研究显示：马立巴韦治疗组的 CMV 转阴率明显优于研究者指定的治疗组（IAT），且副作用较 IAT 组明显降低[27]，由于马立巴韦尚未在中国上市，推荐级别为 2A 类。

9.3 异基因造血干细胞移植后 EB 病毒感染的管理

9.3.1 HSCT 后 EBV 再激活及疾病的监测 [28-33]

	Ⅰ级推荐	Ⅱ级推荐	Ⅲ级推荐
移植前检查	移植前检测供受者 EBV 抗体（2A 类）		移植前检测供受者外周血 EBV-DNA（3 类）
供者选择		血清学阴性患者宜选 EBV 血清学阴性供者（2A 类）	血清学阳性患者宜选 EBV 血清学阳性供者（3 类）
EBV 再激活危险分层	高危患者定义为具有 1 个危险因素：T 细胞去除、供受者 EBV 血清学不合、替代供者、脾切除，二次移植、重度急 / 慢性 GVHD、接受强烈免疫抑制治疗的同胞全相合移植（2A 类）；替代供者移植（无关供者、单倍体供者及脐血移植）		
移植后监测	高危人群定期监测外周血 EBV-DNA[a]（2A 类）		

【注释】

a 外周血 EBV-DNA 监测推荐定量 PCR 检测 EBV-DNA,标本可采用全血、血浆、血清,何种标本最佳尚无定论。阳性阈值目前尚无国际公认标准,需结合本单位情况制订[32]。监测开始时间不晚于 allo-HSCT 后 4 周,如患者具有多个危险因素应提前开始监测;监测频率为每周 1 次,如出现阳性推荐增加监测频率;至少需监测至 allo-HSCT 后 4 个月,对于 T 细胞重建不良的患者(重度急/慢性 GVHD;采用 T 细胞去除(TCD)的单倍体 HSCT;接受过 TCD 治疗;移植后早期出现 EBV 再激活患者)考虑延迟监测时间[32]。

9.3.2 EBV 再激活的预防[32, 34]

	I级推荐	II级推荐	III级推荐
CD20 单抗			预防性应用 CD20 单抗可能降低 EBV-DNA 血症风险,但可能导致持续性全血细胞减少及感染增加(3类)
EBV-CTL			能有效预防 EBV-PTLD 的发生,但受到制备过程的限制(3类)

注:EBV-CTL. EBV 特异性细胞毒性 T 细胞;IVIG. 静脉注射丙种球蛋白。
不推荐用抗病毒药物预防 EBV 再激活,也不推荐应用干扰素或 IVIG 预防。

9.3.3 EBV 血症的抢先治疗 [32, 35-37]

	Ⅰ级推荐	Ⅱ级推荐	Ⅲ级推荐
治疗指征	EBV-DNA 血症 [a]		
抢先治疗方案	CD20 单抗（2A 类） 减量免疫抑制剂（2A 类）		供者或第三方来源 EBV-CTL（3 类），需权衡引起 GVHD 风险

【注释】

a 目前没有公认的开始抢先治疗的外周血 EBV-DNA 阈值，如出现连续 2 次阳性且 EBV-DNA 快速升高或 EBV-DNA 持续阳性，需考虑开始抢先治疗，同时结合单位的临床经验及实验室结果判断[32]。不推荐应用抗病毒药物抢先治疗 EBV 血症。

9.3.4 EBV-PTLD/其他终末器官疾病的治疗 [38-41]

		I 级推荐	II 级推荐	III 级推荐
EBV-PTLD	一线治疗	CD20 单抗（2A 类） 减量免疫抑制剂 + CD20 单抗（2A 类） 不推荐手术、IVIG、抗病毒药物		供者或第三方来源 EBV-CTL（3 类），需权衡引起 GVHD 风险
	二线治疗		EBV-CTL 或 DLI（2A 类）	化疗 +CD20 单抗（2B 类）
CNS-PTLD			CD20 单抗 ± 化疗（2A 类）	静注或鞘注 CD20 单抗 a（3 类） EBV-CTL（3 类），需权衡引起 GVHD 风险 放疗（3 类）
EBV 终末器官疾病		针对累及器官对症支持治疗		CD20 单抗（3 类） 减量免疫抑制剂（3 类）

注：DLI. 供者淋巴细胞输注。

【注释】

a 小样本研究显示鞘注 CD20 单抗对 CNS-PTLD 有效，但剂量和疗程尚需进一步探讨[42-43]。
EBV 疾病的诊断见附录 18。

参考文献

[1] MALLET V, VAN BÖMMEL F, DOERIG C, et al. Management of viral hepatitis in patients with haematological malignancy and in patients undergoing haemopoietic stem cell transplantation: Recommendations of the 5th European Conference on Infections in Leukaemia (ECIL-5). Lancet Infect Dis, 2016, 16 (5): 606-617.

[2] SARMATI L, ANDREONI M, ANTONELLI G, et al. Recommendations for screening, monitoring, prevention, prophylaxis and therapy of hepatitis B virus reactivation in patients with haematologic malignancies and patients who underwent haematologic stem cell transplantation: A position paper. Clin Microbiol Infect, 2017, 23 (12): 935-940.

[3] HWANG JP, FELD JJ, HAMMOND SP, et al. Hepatitis B virus screening and management for patients with cancer prior to therapy: ASCO provisional clinical opinion update. J Clin Oncol, 2020, 38 (31): 3698-3715.

[4] BADEN LR, SWAMINATHAN S, ANGARONE M, et al. Prevention and treatment of cancer-related infections, version 2. 2016, NCCN clinical practice guidelines in oncology. J Natl Compr Canc Netw, 2016, 14 (7): 882-913.

[5] 中华医学会感染病学分会, 中华医学会肝病学分会. 慢性乙型肝炎防治指南 (2019 年版). 临床肝胆病杂志, 2019, 35 (12): 2648-2669.

[6] CORDONNIER C, EINARSDOTTIR S, CESARO S, et al. Vaccination of haemopoietic stem cell transplant recipients: Guidelines of the 2017 European Conference on Infections in Leukaemia (ECIL 7). Lancet Infect

Dis, 2019, 19 (6): e200-e212.

[7] 中国临床肿瘤学会, 中华医学会血液学分会, 中国医师协会肿瘤医师考核委员会, 等. 淋巴瘤免疫化疗乙型肝炎病毒再激活预防和治疗中国专家共识. 中国实用内科杂志, 2014, 34 (1): 32-39.

[8] LJUNGMAN P, DE LA CAMARA R, ROBIN C, et al. Guidelines for the management of cytomegalovirus infection in patients with haematological malignancies and after stem cell transplantation from the 2017 European Conference on Infections in Leukaemia (ECIL 7). Lancet Infect Dis, 2019, 19 (8): e260-e272.

[9] LIN R, LIU Q. Diagnosis and treatment of viral diseases in recipients of allogeneic hematopoietic stem cell transplantation. J Hematol Oncol, 2013, 6: 94.

[10] ZAIA J, BADEN L, BOECKH MJ, et al. Viral disease prevention after hematopoietic cell transplantation. Bone Marrow Transplant, 2009, 44 (8): 471-482.

[11] EMERY V, ZUCKERMAN M, JACKSON G, et al. Management of cytomegalovirus infection in haemopoietic stem cell transplantation. Br J Haematol, 2013, 162 (1): 25-39.

[12] CHEMALY RF, EL HADDAD L, WINSTON DJ, et al. Cytomegalovirus (CMV) cell-mediated immunity and CMV infection after allogeneic hematopoietic cell transplantation: The REACT study. Clin Infect Dis, 2020, 71 (9): 2365-2374.

[13] LJUNGMAN P, DE LA CAMARA R, CORDONNIER C, et al. Management of CMV, HHV-6, HHV-7 and Kaposi-sarcoma herpesvirus (HHV-8) infections in patients with hematological malignancies and after SCT. Bone Marrow Transplant, 2008, 42 (4): 227-240.

[14] MAINOU M, ALAHDAB F, TOBIAN AA, et al. Reducing the risk of transfusion-transmitted cytomegalovirus infection: A systematic review and meta-analysis. Transfusion, 2016, 56 (6Pt 2): 1569-1580.

[15] MARTY FM, LJUNGMAN P, CHEMALY RF, et al. Letermovir prophylaxis for cytomegalo-virus in hematopoietic-cell transplantation. N Engl J Med, 2017, 377 (25): 2433-2444.

[16] HAKKI M, AITKEN SL, DANZIGER-ISAKOV L, et al. American Society for Transplantation and Cellular Therapy Series:#3-prevention of cytomegalovirus infection and disease after hematopoietic cell transplantation. Transplant Cell Ther, 2021, 27 (9): 707-719.

[17] CESARO S, LJUNGMAN P, TRIDELLO G, et al. Trends in the management of cytomegalo virus infection after allogeneic hematopoietic cell transplantation: A survey of the Infectious Diseases Working Pary of EBMT. Bone Marrow Transplant, 2023, 58 (2): 203-208.

[18] BANSAL R, GORDILLO CA, ABRAMOVA R, et al. Extended letermovir administration, be yond day 100, is effective for CMV prophylaxis in patients with graft versus host disease. Transpl Infect Dis, 2021, 23 (2): e13487.

[19] AKAHOSHI Y, KIMURA SI, TADA Y, et al. Cytomegalovirus gastroenteritis in patients with acute graft-versus-host disease. Blood Adv. 2022; 6 (2): 574-584.

[20] MATTES FM, HAINSWORTH EG, GERETTI AM, et al. A randomized, controlled trial comparing ganciclovir to ganciclovir plus foscarnet (each at half dose) for preemptive therapy of cytomegalovirus infection in transplant recipients. J Infect Dis, 2004, 189 (8): 1355-1361.

[21] ZHAO XY, PEI XY, CHANG YJ, et al. First-line therapy with donor-derived human cytomegalovirus (HCMV)-specific T cells reduces persistent hcmv infection by promoting antiviral immunity after allogenic stem cell transplantation. Clin Infect Dis, 2020, 70 (7): 1429-1437.

[22] 刘启发. 我如何管理造血干细胞移植后巨细胞病毒感染. 中华血液学杂志, 2017, 38 (11): 916-919.

[23] ARIZA-HEREDIA EJ, NESHER L, CHEMALY RF. Cytomegalovirus diseases after hematopoietic stem cell transplantation: A mini-review. Cancer Lett, 2014, 342 (1): 1-8.

[24] YONG MK, SHIGLE TL, KIM YJ, et al. American Society for Transplantation and Cellular Therapy Series:#4-cytomegalovirus treatment and management of resistant or refractory infections after hematopoietic cell transplantation. Transplant Cell Ther, 2021, 27 (12): 957-967.

[25] BHUTANI D, DYSON G, MANASA R, et al. Incidence, risk factors, and outcome of cytomegalovirus viremia and gastroenteritis in patients with gastrointestinal graft-versus-host disease. Biol Blood Marrow Transplant, 2015, 21 (1): 159-164.

[26] SEO S, RENAUD C, KUYPERS JM, et al. Idiopathic pneumonia syndrome after hematopoietic cell transplantation: evidence of occult infectious etiologies. Blood, 2015, 125 (24): 3789-3797.

[27] AVERY RK, ALAIN S, ALEXANDER BD, et al. Maribavir for refractory cytomegalovirus infections with or without resistance post-transplant: Results from a phase 3 randomized clinical trial. Clin Infect Dis, 2022, 75 (4): 690-701.

[28] LIN R, WANG Y, HUANG F, et al. Two dose levels of rabbit antithymocyte globulin as graft-versus-host disease prophylaxis in haploidentical stem cell transplantation: A multicenter randomized study. BMC Med, 2019, 17 (1): 156.

[29] UHLIN M, WIKELL H, SUNDIN M, et al. Risk factors for Epstein-Barr virus-related post-transplant lymphoproliferative disease after allogeneic hematopoietic stem cell transplantation. Haematologica, 2014, 99 (2): 346-352.

[30] LANDGREN O, GILBERT ES, RIZZO JD, et al. Risk factors for lymphoproliferative disorders after allogeneic hematopoietic cell transplantation. Blood, 2009, 113 (20): 4992-5001.

[31] SUNDIN M, LE BLANC K, RINGDÉN O, et al. The role of HLA mismatch, splenectomy and recipient Epstein-Barr virus seronegativity as risk factors in post-transplant lymphoproliferative disorder following allogeneic hematopoietic stem cell transplantation. Haematologica, 2006, 91 (8): 1059-1067.

[32] STYCZYNSKI J, VAN DER VELDEN W, FOX CP, et al. Management of Epstein-Barr virus infections and post-transplant lymphoproliferative disorders in patients after allogeneic hematopoietic stem cell transplantation: Sixth European Conference on Infections in Leukemia (ECIL-6) guidelines. Haematologica, 2016, 101 (7): 803-811.

[33] KANAKRY JA, KASAMON YL, BOLAÑOS-MEADE J, et al. Absence of post-transplantation lymphoproliferative disorder after allogeneic blood or marrow transplantation using post-transplantation cyclophosphamide as graft-

[34] DOMINIETTO A, TEDONE E, SORACCO M, et al. In vivo B-cell depletion with rituximab for alternative donor hemopoietic SCT. Bone Marrow Transplant, 2012, 47 (1): 101-106.

[35] LIU Q, XUAN L, LIU H, et al. Molecular monitoring and stepwise preemptive therapy for Epstein-Barr virus viremia after allogeneic stem cell transplantation. Am J Hematol, 2013, 88 (7): 550-555.

[36] WORTH A, CONYERS R, COHEN J, et al. Pre-emptive rituximab based on viraemia and T cell reconstitution: A highly effective strategy for the prevention of Epstein-Barr virus-associated lymphoproliferative disease following stem cell transplantation. Br J Haematol, 2011, 155 (3): 377-385.

[37] VAN ESSER JW, NIESTERS HG, VAN DER HOLT B, et al. Prevention of Epstein-Barr virus-lymphoproliferative disease by molecular monitoring and preemptive rituximab in high-risk patients after allogeneic stem cell transplantation. Blood, 2002, 99 (12): 4364-4369.

[38] STYCZYNSKI J, GIL L, TRIDELLO G, et al. Response to rituximab-based therapy and risk factor analysis in Epstein-Barr virus-related lymphoproliferative disorder after hematopoietic stem cell transplant in children and adults: A study from the Infectious Diseases Working Party of the European Group for Blood and Marrow Transplantation. Clin Infect Dis, 2013, 57 (6): 794-802.

[39] XU LP, ZHANG CL, MO XD, et al. Epstein-Barr virus-related post-transplantation lymphoproliferative disorder after unmanipulated human leukocyte antigen haploidentical hematopoietic stem cell tra-nsplantation: Incidence, risk factors, treatment, and clinical outcomes. Biol Blood Marrow Transplant, 2015, 21 (12): 2185-2191.

[40] LIU QF, LING YW, FAN ZP, et al. Epstein-Barr virus (EBV) load in cerebrospinal fluid and peripheral blood of patients with EBV-associated central nervous system diseases after allogeneic hematopoietic stem cell transplantation. Transpl Infect Dis, 2013, 15 (4): 379-392.

[41] JIANG X, XU L, ZHANG Y, et al. Rituximab-based treatments followed by adoptive cellular immunotherapy for

biopsy-proven EBV-associated post-transplant lymphoproliferative disease in recipients of allogeneic hematopoietic stem cell transplantation. Oncoimmunology, 2016, 5 (5): e1139274.

[42] WU M, SUN J, ZHANG Y, et al. Intrathecal rituximab for EBV-associated post-transplant lymphoproliferative disorder with central nervous system involvement unresponsive to intravenous rituximab-based treatments: A prospective study. Bone Marrow Transplant, 2016, 51 (3): 456-458.

[43] SWERDLOW SH, CAMPO E, PILERI SA, et al. The 2016 revision of the World Health Organization classification of lymphoid neoplasms. Blood, 2016, 127 (20): 2375-2390.

10 异基因造血干细胞移植后白血病/骨髓增生异常综合征复发的监测、预防、治疗

10.1 移植后复发的监测

10.1.1 常用 MRD 检测方法

常用检测方法	I 级推荐	II 级推荐	III 级推荐
多参数流式细胞术（MFC）	检测白血病相关免疫表型（LAIP）或有别于正常的表型（different from normal，DfN），灵敏度 $10^{-4} \sim 10^{-3}$（2A 类）[1]		
染色体		G 显带、R 显带和/或荧光原位杂交（FISH），灵敏度 10^{-2}（2A 类）	

常用 MRD 检测方法(续)

常用检测方法	I 级推荐	II 级推荐	III 级推荐
RT-qPCR		检测特异的白血病相关基因或基因突变,证据充分靶点: *NPM1*, *CBFB-MYH11*, *RUNX1-RUNX1T1* 灵敏度 $10^{-5}\sim10^{-4}$(2A 类)	证据欠缺靶点: *KMT2A-MLLT3*(即 *MLL-AF9*),*DEK-NUP214*,*BCR-ABL1*,*WT1* 灵敏度 $10^{-5}\sim10^{-4}$
供受者嵌合状态的检测		STR-PCR 或 FISH(性别不合移植),灵敏度 1%~5%(2A 类)	
二代测序(NGS)			除胚系突变和克隆性造血突变(DAT)以外的所有的体细胞突变均具有潜在 MRD 的预后判断价值,灵敏度 $10^{-4}\sim10^{-2}$(3 类)

常用 MRD 检测方法（续）

常用检测方法	Ⅰ级推荐	Ⅱ级推荐	Ⅲ级推荐
数字 PCR（dPCR）			特异性突变和白血病融合基因：NPM1 突变和（CBF）-AML 融合基因灵敏度 $10^{-4} \sim 10^{-3}$（3类）

【注释】

1. MRD 监测的意义　MRD 的监测应该贯穿移植的前中后，并应在移植后尽早监测 MRD 来预测患者预后。多种 MRD 监测手段的联合应用可以提高对移植后复发预测的灵敏度。移植前 MRD 监测可为患者的预后及移植后复发风险评估提供依据。

2. PCR 检测的分子学标志　AML 患者 MRD 常用的靶基因包括特异分子生物学标志 [*TEL-AML1*、*BCR-ABL*、*RUNX1-RUNX1T1*（*AML1-ETO*）、*CBFβ-MYH11*、*NPM1*、*MLL* 重排等] 和非特异标志（*IgH* 重排、*WT1* 等）。ALL 患者 MRD 常用的靶基因包括 *BCR-ABL* 和非特异标志（IgH 重排）。

3. DAT　指 *DNMT3A*、*ASXL1* 和 *TET2* 突变，这三个基因突变都是与克隆性造血相关的突变，因此不能做为 MRD 的监测指标。

4. 监测频率　AML 和 ALL 一般建议在移植后 +1、+2、+3、+4、+6、+9、+12、+18、+24、+36、+48、+60 个月检测骨髓形态学、MRD 和嵌合状态，必要时增加检测频度。出现 MRD 时，建议 2 周内复查以明确是否有复发趋势。移植后一旦复发，应该完善骨髓形态、免疫分型、融合基因和细胞来源的检查；CML 患者融合基因检测：建议每 3 个月 1 次，共 2 年；随后每 6 个月 1 次，共 3 年。进行骨髓或外周血的 PCR 监测，达到完全细胞遗传学反应（CCyR）且融合基因检测持续阴性者按上述频率持续监测，allo-HSCT 后及早发现 BCR-ABL1 转录本有助于在出现复发之前识别可能需要抢先治疗的患者。骨髓染色体核型分析或 FISH：建议每 3 个月 1 次，共 2 年；随后每 6 个月 1 次，共 3 年。

5. HLA loss 尚无标准化监测方法，文献推荐应用 NGS 或者定量 PCR。检测 HLA Loss 的时机为患者出现血液学复发时。

10.1.2 判定 MRD 阳性的标准

检测方法	I级推荐	II级推荐	III级推荐
MFC	连续2次阳性,且间隔10~14天(2A类)		
PCR 监测		WT1阳性阈值应根据各单位所采用的检测技术和结果进行设定,WT1连续2次阳性,且间隔10~14天(2A类) 对于NPM1、RUNX1-RUNX1T1、CBFβ-MYH11、DEK-NUP214将MRD阳性定为>1%(2A类)	
STR-PCR 或 FISH		动态监测STR(2A类)	
NGS	实验室NGS检测灵敏度及病理意义精准解读是目前阻碍NGS-MRD在常规诊断中实施的主要问题。目前尚无具体的推荐来保证NGS在不同实验室之间的标准化和可比性(1A类)		动态监测骨髓NGS-MRD有助于判断移植预后:所有移植前和移植后1个月突变均持续阳性的AML患者,与移植后更高的复发率和更差的总体生存率显著相关(3类)[2]

【注释】

1. MFC　仍然采用 ELWP 的 0.1%（AML）以及 0.01%（ALL）。

2. PCR　北京大学人民医院报道 WT1 阳性的界值为 0.6%，儿童为 1.5% 左右[3]，其他中心根据各自实验室的标准进行阈值设定。不同病种的 MRD 阳性标准如下。Ph+ALL：①移植后 *BCR-ABL* 融合基因未转阴；②连续 2 次（间隔小于 1 个月）复查的结果未降低；③移植后任何时间点高于 1% 或移植后 BCR-ABL 由阴性转为阳性。CML：①移植后 1 个月 *BCR-ABL* 融合基因比基线水平未下降 2 个对数值且连续 2 次（间隔小于 2 个月）复查的结果未降低；②移植后 3 个月未达到 MMR（比基线水平下降 3 个 log）；③移植后 BCR-ABL 连续 2 次检测（间隔 2 个月内）由阴转阳或上升 1 个 log。伴 RUNX1-RUNX1T1 白血病：①移植后 1、2、3 个月 RUNX1-RUNX1T1 较基线水平下降小于 3 个对数级；②移植后 RUNX1-RUNX1T1 高于 0.4%。伴 CBFβ-MYH11 白血病：移植后与基线相比下降小于 3 个 log。其他类型白血病（MLL、TLS-ERG、E2A-PBX1、SIL-TAL1、ETV6-RUNX1）：检测到超过 0 则认为 MRD 阳性。

3. STR 或 FISH 显示嵌合体受者比例增加　当采用嵌合状态判定干预指征时，尚无统一意见，动态监测 STR 有助于判断疾病复发并指导免疫调节治疗的时机和疗效。系列特异性 STR 可提高检测的灵敏度。

4. *NPM1* 突变是目前监测移植后 MRD 有效的指标　在移植后采用等位基因特异性寡核苷酸聚合酶链式反应（ASO-PCR）动态检测骨髓中 NPM1 突变，移植后 NPM1 突变水平增加 10% 以上与移植后复发、不良预后相关[4]。

10.2 移植后复发的预防

10.2.1 AML 移植后复发的预防

预防策略	Ⅰ级推荐	Ⅱ级推荐	Ⅲ级推荐
供者选择		MRD 阳性的高危 AML 患者或者拥有年轻子女的老年 AML 患者优先选择单倍型移植（2A 类）	
预处理方案改进		NR 患者预处理应用低剂量 DAC 联合改良 BUCY（2A 类）	预处理加入新药（3 类）
免疫治疗	提前减停免疫抑制剂、预防性或抢先性 DLI[5]（2A 类）		加用干扰素 -α、IL-2、乌苯美司等（3 类）
靶向药物	FLT3 抑制剂索拉非尼（1A 类）		
去甲基化药物	地西他滨（DAC）联合 G-CSF[6]（1A 类）、阿扎胞苷（AZA）巩固维持[7-8]（2A 类）		

【注释】

1. **预防治疗** 是指针对移植前处于复发/难治状态的高危患者在出现细胞遗传学/分子（生物）学复发前采取的措施。

2. **供体选择** 针对移植前形态学缓解 MRD 阳性 AML 患者，单倍体移植与同胞全相合相比，无白血病生存率显著更高，提示对于移植前 MRD 阳性 AML 患者，单倍体移植预后更佳[9]。

3. **预处理加入新药**，新药应具备更强抗肿瘤活性和/或更低毒性。

4. **免疫抑制剂减停** 同胞 HLA 全相合移植 60 天内、非血缘脐血移植 60 天内、单倍型移植 100 天内减停免疫抑制剂需谨慎。

5. **DLI 预防性治疗** ①输注时机，如果移植后无 GVHD，早期应用（+30 ~ +120 天）。②输注细胞，可以采用单采的供体淋巴细胞或者改良 DLI，G-CSF 动员后的供者细胞；回输剂量根据不同移植方式，移植后时间长短，肿瘤负荷水平决定输注剂量。以剂量递增方式输注，新鲜或冻存的 MNC 均可，建议移植时冻存备用。③ DLI 相关 GVHD 预防，根据本中心的经验，决定是否预防。北京大学人民医院推荐继续原有 CsA，同胞 HLA 相合 DLI 后应用 CsA 不少于 4 周；单倍型 DLI 后 CsA 应用不少于 6 周，至少用到移植后 100 天。MTX 预防 GVHD，DLI 后 1、4、8 天各给药 1 次，以后 10mg 每周 1 次共 4~6 次。

10.2.2 ALL 移植后复发的预防

	I 级推荐	II 级推荐	III 级推荐
移植方式选择	MRD 阳性患者优先选择单倍型移植（2A 类）	①无关供者移植（推荐选择 MUD，无 MUD 的情况下可选择 MMUD）[10]（2A 类） ②脐带血干细胞移植[11]（2A 类）	
预处理方案调整	TBI 联合 CTX（2A 类）	TBI/Cy 联合 VP-16[12]（2A 类）	新药（2B 类）
靶向药物治疗	Ph+ ALL： ①预防性应用 TKI 大于 1 年，定期监测 BCR-ABL，若为阴性或转阴则停药，继续监测，若为阳性则按抢先治疗处理（2A 类） ②血液学缓解患者，BCR-ABL 为阴性也应预防性应用 TKI（2A 类）		Ph-ALL MRD 阳性患者移植前采用贝林妥欧使 MRD 转阴（2B 类） B-ALL：奥加伊妥珠单抗治疗（2B 类）

ALL 移植后复发的预防（续）

	I 级推荐	II 级推荐	III 级推荐
免疫治疗	Ph-ALL：预防性应用 DLI（可选 mDLI）（2A 类）	提前减停免疫抑制剂（2A 类）	免疫调节剂治疗（3 类）
其他			MPAL：CAR-T 治疗桥接异基因造血干细胞移植[13]（3 类）

【注释】

1. 预处理方案　全身照射（TBI）剂量：12Gy 分 6 次照射。

2. TKI　伊马替尼的起始剂量为 400mg/d，无效后进入抢先治疗；也可以参考移植前疗效和基因突变情况选用其他类型的 TKI。

3. 贝林妥欧单抗（blinatumomab）是一种 CD3/CD19 的双特异性抗体，可以特异性结合 B 细胞表面的 CD19 与 T 细胞表面的 CD3 受体，目前贝林妥欧单抗治疗 Ph-ALL 的疗效已得到证实，能够使患者 MRD 转阴，在深度缓解的状态下接受移植[14]。

4. 减停免疫抑制剂的说明　同胞全相合移植、非亲缘脐血移植不推荐在 60 天内减停免疫抑制剂、单倍型移植不推荐在 100 天内减停免疫抑制剂，在有活动性的 GVHD 的前提下不推荐提前减停。

5. 奥加伊妥珠单抗为靶向 CD22 的抗体偶联药物（ADC），在 CD22 低表达或不表达时不推荐使用，应用过程中需要关注肝小静脉闭塞病（VOD）的发生。

10.2.3　MDS 移植后复发的预防

	I 级推荐	II 级推荐	III 级推荐
免疫抑制剂	酌情减停（2A 类）		
化疗		减低剂量去甲基化治疗（2A 类）	
其他			
预处理方案			地西他滨 +BUCY2 强化预处理方案（3 类）

【注释】

1. 对于移植前经强化化疗或去甲基化药物治疗后未达 CR、移植前外周血原始细胞比例 >3% 及有基因（*TP53*、*EZH2*、*ETV6*、*RUNX1*、*ASXL1*）突变的 MDS 患者采取维持治疗以预防复发。

2. 免疫调节治疗　在没有 GVHD 的情况下，①提前减停免疫抑制剂（+100 天前）：+30 天开始减少 MMF，+60~90 天减少环孢素；②预防性 DLI 治疗：如果患者无 GVHD 发生或明显复发，可建议在 +100 天后或停用免疫抑制药 1 个月后进行预防性 DLI 治疗。

3. 减低剂量去甲基化治疗　①阿扎胞苷 $32\text{mg/m}^2 \times 5$ 天，每月一次；②地西他滨 $5\sim10\text{mg/m}^2 \times 5$ 天，每月一次；如果可以耐受，+60 天开始，疗程为 12~24 个月。

4. AZA 联合 DLI 是目前用于治疗移植后复发高危 MDS 的有效方案。

10.2.4 CML 移植后复发的预防

移植前为进展期(AP 及 BP)且移植后 *BCR/ABL1* 融合基因持续阴性的患者需 TKI 治疗至少 1 年(2A 类),治疗起始时间从移植后第 3 个月开始,TKI 药物的选择取决于移植前对 TKI 治疗反应、预期毒性以及 BCR/ABL1 激酶区突变情况。对于移植后没有干预治疗的患者,除监测融合基因外,也要进行微小残留病变的监测。

突变类型	药物选择
V299L	尼洛替尼、博纳替尼
T315A	尼洛替尼或博舒替尼、博纳替尼、伊马替尼(如果是在达沙替尼治疗中出现的)
F317L/V/I/C	尼洛替尼、博纳替尼、博舒替尼
Y253H	达沙替尼或博舒替尼、博纳替尼
E255K/V	达沙替尼或博舒替尼、博纳替尼
F359V/C/I	达沙替尼或博舒替尼、博纳替尼
T315I	博纳替尼或奥马西他辛或奥雷巴替尼以及临床试验
任意其他突变	博纳替尼、达沙替尼、尼洛替尼、博舒替尼

10.3 移植后复发的抢先治疗

10.3.1 AML 移植后复发的抢先治疗

抢先策略	Ⅰ级推荐	Ⅱ级推荐	Ⅲ级推荐
免疫抑制剂	酌情减停		
靶向药物			如 FLT3 抑制剂（3 类）
细胞免疫治疗	DLI[15]（2A 类）		CAR-T（3 类）
干扰素		IFN-α[16-18]	

【注释】

1. 抢先治疗指对移植后出现细胞遗传学/分子（生物）学复发、未达血液学复发的患者采取的措施。干预时机或适用人群：参考 MRD 阳性标准即抢先治疗的指征。
2. 减停免疫抑制剂　根据移植后 MRD 发生时间和 GVHD 情况决定。+100 天内减停需谨慎。

10.3.2 ALL 移植后复发的抢先治疗

	Ⅰ级推荐	Ⅱ级推荐	Ⅲ级推荐
免疫抑制剂的调整		减停免疫抑制剂（2A 类）	
靶向药物	Ph+ALL：TKI（2A 类）	Ph-ALL：入组临床试验或者选择新的靶向药物（2A 类）	
免疫治疗	肿瘤消减治疗 +DLI（可选择 mDLI）（2A 类）		单独 DLI 治疗（3 类） blinatumomab[19]（3 类） CAR-T、NK 细胞治疗等（3 类）
干扰素治疗			IFN-α-2b（2B 类）
其他			

【注释】

1. 减停免疫抑制剂　根据移植后 MRD+ 时间和 GVHD 情况决定。+100 天内减停需谨慎。
2. 靶向药物选择：若存在 ABL 激酶区突变，可根据突变位点选择合适 TKI。① *Y253H*、*E255K/V*、

F359C/V/I：达沙替尼；② *F317L/V/I/C*、*V299L*、*T315A*：尼洛替尼；③两者均耐药，可以考虑奥雷巴替尼，目前已在国内上市，博纳替尼抑或入组临床试验，博纳替尼国外经验疗效确切，我国尚未上市。

3. 消减肿瘤治疗 +DLI（可选择 mDLI） ①消减肿瘤治疗方案根据患者的体能状态、有无合并症、白血病生物学特征、治疗靶点以及既往化疗敏感方案，选择合适的治疗方案；②输注细胞及 GVHD 的预防见预防措施。

4. DLI 前首先考虑减停免疫抑制剂，减停时机 ① +2~+90 天：维持原有 CsA，予化疗 +DLI；②>+90 天：第一次 MRD（+）时即停用 CsA，观察两周，若 GVHD（−）而 MRD（+）予化疗 + DLI，若 GVHD（−）且 MRD（−）可用 IFN-α。活动性 GVHD 不推荐进行 DLI，建议在 DLI 后 1、2、3、4、5、6、7、12 个月评估 MRD，之后每 6 个月评估一次，根据 MRD 及 GVHD 状态调整治疗方案。

5. 干扰素治疗 使用 IFN-α-2b 治疗时，如果：①患者不能耐受治疗；②发生Ⅲ度或更高级别的 GVHD；③经过 1 个月以上的治疗后病情没有得到控制并有进展时，应终止治疗。

10.3.3 MDS 移植后复发的抢先治疗

治疗策略	Ⅰ级推荐	Ⅱ级推荐	Ⅲ级推荐
免疫抑制剂	停用免疫抑制剂（2A 类）		
化疗	去甲基化药物（2A 类）		
免疫治疗			干扰素（3 类）

【注释】

1. 抢先治疗 对于移植前达 CR，移植后 MRD 检测阳性或者供者嵌合度降低（与 MRD 无关）的患者进行抢先治疗。

2. 免疫调节 在没有 GVHD 的情况下，①提前减停免疫抑制剂（+100 天之前）；②+100 天后抢先 DLI 治疗。

3. 去甲基化药物 ①阿扎胞苷：阿扎胞苷 $75mg/m^2 \times 7$ 天，皮下注射，每月 1 次；②地西他滨：地西他滨 $20mg/m^2 \times 5$ 天~10 天，每月 1 次，但会出现明显的血液学毒性；在同种异体移植后早期（<100 天）出现白细胞减少或血小板减少的情况下减低剂量。如果出现肾功能不全、Ⅳ度肝毒性或出现 GVHD 或严重恶化，应停止治疗。在 MRD 阳性或供者嵌合度降低后尽快开始治疗，根据反应如果可以耐受，应持续 12~24 个月。

4. 北京大学血液病研究所的前瞻性临床研究显示，MRD 阳性患者应用抢先干预性干扰素治疗与干预性 DLI（化疗+DLI）疗效相当[20]。重组人干扰素 α，2~3 次/周，皮下注射 6 个周期，≥16 岁患者，每次 3MU（百万单位），<16 岁每次 3MU/m²（上限 3MU）。可酌情延长干扰素 α 的治疗时间，若出现严重 GVHD、严重感染、≥3 度毒性，则停用干扰素。

10.3.4 CML 移植后 MRD 阳性患者的抢先治疗

治疗策略	Ⅰ级推荐	Ⅱ级推荐	Ⅲ级推荐
免疫抑制剂	减停免疫抑制剂		
化疗		高三尖杉酯碱	
免疫治疗	DLI（2A 类）	干扰素	
靶向治疗	TKI（2A 类）		
其他		临床试验	

【注释】

1. MRD 阳性患者，应检测 ABL 激酶区是否存在突变，依照检测结果选择 TKI 治疗。同时取决于既往 TKI 治疗的反应、耐受性。

2. 奥马西他辛已经证实可以对多种 TKI 耐药的 AP-CML 患者包括携带 *T315I* 突变的患者有效[21]，其用法为 1.25mg/m²，2 次/d，皮下注射，d1~14，每 28 天为一疗程。

10.4 移植后复发的治疗

10.4.1 AML 移植后复发的治疗

治疗策略	Ⅰ级推荐	Ⅱ级推荐	Ⅲ级推荐
免疫抑制剂	停用免疫抑制剂（2A 类）*		
化疗		根据患者体能状态、合并症、肿瘤负荷、既往治疗有效方案选择相应治疗方案	
免疫治疗	建议化疗 + DLI*（2A 类）		IFN-α 活化 DLI[22]、CAR-T 治疗[23]、供者 NK 细胞治疗（3类）CD38 CAR-T[24]、CD19 CAR-T[25] 和 CLL1 CAR-T[26] 治疗（3类）
靶向治疗		FLT3 抑制剂（2A 类）	如 Bcl-2 抑制剂、临床试验（3类）
去甲基化药物		地西他滨、阿扎胞苷联合其他治疗方案（2A 类）	
二次移植		二次移植（2A 类）	

*.有条件的单位应在复发时先检测 HLA Loss。

【注释】

1. AML 移植后复发　如果为 HLA-loss 型复发,停用免疫抑制剂和 DLI 治疗并不能增强 GVL 效应,对复发的治疗是无效的[27]。

2. 化疗方案选择　根据原始细胞数、既往用药史选择既往有效或目前治疗单位常用的方案,如阿糖胞苷 + 阿克拉霉素（AA）或阿糖胞苷 + 高三尖杉酯碱（HA）,也可选择其他新药如去甲基化药物等。DLI 方案：化疗药物停止 2~3 个半衰期后输注；北京大学血液病研究所输注 G-CSF 动员后的外周血造血干细胞有核细胞剂量为 1×10^8/kg；也可选择递增式输注等方式。

3. DLI 相关 GVHD 预防　依供者类型和既往 GVHD 情况选用 CsA 或 MTX,同胞 HLA 相合者 DLI 后应用 MTX 共 4 周,每周 1 次,每次 10mg；单倍型移植患者,如复发前无重度 GVHD,应用 CsA 3 周,之后无 GVHD 开始减量继之以 MTX 3 周,用法如上；如复发前曾有重度 GVHD,应用 CsA 6 周,4 周时无 GVHD 即开始减量,至 6 周停药。若为同胞 HLA 全相合移植,递增式 DLI 不一定常规作 GVHD 预防。

4. Bcl-2 抑制剂　venetoclax 目前常与其他药物联合应用,如去甲基化药、低剂量阿糖胞苷和挽救性化疗方案。

5. 二次移植　应根据复发时间早晚、上述治疗后 MRD 是否转阴,并结合患者身体状况、个人意愿决定是否进行。二次移植时应考虑 HLA-loss 复发的患者不能再次选择原供者,需更换其他合适的供者。

6. 髓外复发　目前无推荐方案。除上述全身治疗外,可采用局部放疗,另外采用腰椎穿刺联合鞘注的方法预防及治疗 CNSL。

10.4.2 ALL 移植后复发的治疗

治疗	Ⅰ级推荐	Ⅱ级推荐	Ⅲ级推荐
免疫调整		停用免疫抑制剂（WIS）（2A 类）	
靶向药物	Ph+ALL：TKI 治疗（2A 类） Ph-B-ALL：联合分子靶向治疗或者联合免疫靶向治疗	Ph-ALL：可入组临床试验（2A 类）	
免疫治疗	化疗+DLI（可选择 mDLI）（2A 类） B-ALL：CD19 CAR-T 细胞治疗[28]（2A 类）	B-ALL：序贯使用（CD19/CD22）CAR-T 治疗[29]（2A 类） Ph+ALL：贝林妥欧单抗 ± TKI 治疗[30] Ph-ALL：贝林妥欧单抗（2A 类）	其他免疫治疗联合 mDLI（3 类） T-ALL：CD7 CAR-T 治疗[31]（3 类） B-ALL：奥加伊妥珠单抗治疗[32]（2B 类）

ALL 移植后复发的治疗（续）

治疗	Ⅰ级推荐	Ⅱ级推荐	Ⅲ级推荐
化疗	氟达拉滨 + 蒽环类药物或以氟达拉滨为基础的方案（2A 类）		
二次移植			如化疗或靶向治疗有效，可行二次移植（2B 类）
其他	临床试验		
髓外白血病复发的治疗	CNSL：鞘内注射化疗药物/全脑加全脊髓放疗（2A 类）		EMR（除 CNSL）：全身治疗联合或不联合 DLI 或单独局部治疗（3 类）

【注释】

1. 免疫调整　移植后复发仅停用免疫抑制剂很难达到完全缓解，针对少数肿瘤负荷低、较惰性的白血病可能有效[33]。复发但未发生 GVHD 的患者可以考虑停用免疫抑制剂（WIS）。

2. 免疫治疗　化疗 +DLI（可选择 mDLI），输注时间、输注细胞及 GVHD 的预防见预防措施。

3. 靶向药物治疗　使用 TKI 治疗期间连续监测 BCR-ABL 均转阴，TKI 至少应用 1 年，若持续不转阴或转阴后再次转阳,进行 ABL 激酶区突变检查后决定是否更换 TKI(更换方案见抢先治疗)。

4. 髓外复发的治疗　局部治疗包括手术切除、鞘内注射和局部放疗,全身治疗包括化疗、DLI 和二次移植,多数研究显示,单纯局部治疗往往伴随之后包括髓内的全面复发,故推荐进行全身治疗 ± DLI 进行治疗,鞘注化疗应掌握时机,推荐在外周血没有原始细胞,血细胞计数安全后行腰椎穿刺。药物可选择 MTX 10~15mg/ 次 + 地塞米松(两联)或 MTX+Ara-C 30~50mg/ 次 + 地塞米松(三联)。鞘内注射次数一般应达 6 次以上,高危组患者应达 12 次以上。鞘内注射频率不超过 2 次 / 周,放疗一般在缓解后巩固化疗期或维持治疗时进行。头颅放疗剂量 2.0~2.4Gy,脊髓放疗剂量 1.8~2.0Gy,分次完成。此外,奥加伊妥珠单抗对 CNSL 治疗也有更好的效果[34]

10.4.3　MDS 移植后复发的治疗

治疗策略	Ⅰ级推荐	Ⅱ级推荐	Ⅲ级推荐
二次移植	二次移植(2A 类)		
免疫治疗	化疗联合 DLI 或 DLI(2A 类)		
靶向治疗			IDH2 抑制剂 Enasidenib(3 类)

【注释】

1. 化疗联合 DLI　①治疗前应确认供受者嵌合状态是否为供者型;②化疗方案选择:阿糖胞苷 +

阿克拉霉素（AA）或阿糖胞苷+高三尖杉酯碱（HA）；③ DLI：化疗药物停止 2~3 个半衰期后输注。

2. 二次移植　没有证据支持二次移植换用另一个供者可进一步获益。

3. 新型靶向治疗　*IDH2* 突变蛋白抑制剂 Enasidenib 可以诱导 *IDH2* 突变的 MDS 患者血液学甚至分子水平缓解。另外，APR-246 可用于治疗 *Tp53* 阳性 MDS。

10.4.4　CML 移植后复发的治疗

停用免疫抑制剂，可考虑 TKI 联合或不联合 DLI（TKI 的选择取决于先前的治疗，BCR-ABL1 突变状态以及移植后的并发症）或奥马西他辛或临床试验（2A 类）。

【注释】

达沙替尼用于治疗 allo-HSCT 后髓外复发可能有效，包括 CNSL 的复发[35]。

参考文献

[1] DOHNER H, WEI AH, APPELBAUM FR, et al. Diagnosis and management of AML in adults: 2022 recommendations from an international expert panel on behalf of the ELN. Blood, 2022, 140 (12): 1345-1377.

[2] KIM HJ, KIM Y, KANG D, et al. Prognostic value of measurable residual disease monitoring by next-generation sequencing before and after allogeneic hematopoietic cell transplantation in acute myeloid leukemia. Blood Cancer J, 2021, 11 (6): 109.

[3] ZHAO XS, YAN CH, LIU DH, et al. Combined use of WT1 and flow cytometry monitoring can promote sensitivity of predicting relapse after allogeneic HSCT without affecting specificity. Ann Hematol, 2013, 92 (8): 1111-1119.

[4] SHAYEGI N, KRAMER M, BORNHÄUSER M, et al. The level of residual disease based on mutant NPM1 is an independent prognostic factor for relapse and survival in AML. Blood, 2013, 122 (1): 83-92.

[5] SCHMID C, LABOPIN M, SCHAAP N, et al. Prophylactic donor lymphocyte infusion after allogeneic stem cell transplantation in acute leukaemia-a matched pair analysis by the Acute Leukaemia Working Party of EBMT. Br J Haematol, 2019, 184 (5): 782-787.

[6] GAO L, ZHANG Y, WANG S, et al. Effect of rhG-CSF combined with decitabine prophylaxis on relapse of patients with high-risk MRD-negative AML after HSCT: An open-label, multicenter, randomized controlled trial. J Clin Oncol, 2020, 38 (36): 4249-4259.

[7] MA Y, QU C, DAI H, et al. Maintenance therapy with decitabine after allogeneic hematopoietic stem cell transplantation to prevent relapse of high-risk acute myeloid leukemia. Bone Marrow Transplant, 2020, 55 (6): 1206-1208.

[8] DE LIMA M, GIRALT S, THALL PF, et al. Maintenance therapy with low-dose azacitidine after allogeneic hematopoietic stem cell transplantation for recurrent acute myelogenous leukemia or myelodysplastic syndrome: A dose and schedule finding study. Cancer, 2010, 116 (23): 5420-5431.

[9] CHANG YJ, WANG Y, LIU YR, et al. Haploidentical allograft is superior to matched sibling donor allograft in eradicating pre-transplantation minimal residual disease of AML patients as determined by multiparameter flow cytometry: A retrospective and prospective analysis. J Hematol Oncol, 2017, 10 (1): 134.

[10] KINDWALL-KELLER TL, BALLEN KK. Alternative donor graft sources for adults with hematologic malignancies: A donor for all patients in 2017. Oncologist, 2017, 22 (9): 1125-1134.

[11] WIEDUWILT MJ, METHENY L, ZHANG MJ, et al. Haploidentical vs sibling, unrelated, or cord blood hematopoietic cell transplantation for acute lymphoblastic leukemia. Blood Adv, 2022, 6 (1): 339-357.

[12] SHIGEMATSU A, TANAKA J, SUZUKI R, et al. Outcome of medium-dose VP-16/CY/TBI superior to CY/TBI as a conditioning regimen for allogeneic stem cell transplantation in adult patients with acute lymphoblastic leukemia. Int J Hematol, 2011, 94 (5): 463-471.

[13] KONG D, QU C, DAI H, et al. CAR-T therapy bridging to allogeneic HSCT provides durable molecular remission of Ph+ mixed phenotype acute leukaemia with minimal residual disease. Br J Haematol, 2020, 191 (2): e47-e49.

[14] GÖKBUGET N, DOMBRET H, BONIFACIO M, et al. Blinatumomab for minimal residual disease in adults with B-cell precursor acute lymphoblastic leukemia. Blood, 2018, 131 (14): 1522-1531.

[15] CASTAGNA L, SARINA B, BRAMANTI S, et al. Donor lymphocyte infusion after allogeneic stem cell transplantation. Transfus Apher Sci, 2016, 54 (3): 345-355.

[16] LIN XJ, DAI HP, WANG AJ, et al. Effects of preemptive interferon-α monotherapy in acute leukemia patients with relapse tendency after allogeneic hematopoietic stem cell transplantation: A case-control study. Ann Hematol, 2018, 97 (11): 2195-2204.

[17] SHEN MZ, ZHANG XH, XU LP, et al. Preemptive interferon-α therapy could protect against relapse and improve survival of acute myeloid leukemia patients after allogeneic hematopoietic stem cell transplantation: Long-term results of two registry studies. Front Immunol, 2022, 13: 757002.

[18] FAN S, SHEN MZ, ZHANG XH, et al. Preemptive immunotherapy for minimal residual disease in patients with t (8; 21) acute myeloid leukemia after allogeneic hematopoietic stem cell transplantation. Front Oncol, 2021, 11: 773394.

[19] GABALLA MR, BANERJEE PP, MILTON DR, et al. Blinatumomab maintenance after allogeneic hematopoietic cell transplantation for B-lineage acute lymphoblastic leukemia. Blood, 2021013290.

[20] MO X, ZHANG X, XU L, et al. Minimal residual disease-directed immunotherapy for high-risk myelodysplastic syndrome after allogeneic hematopoietic stem cell transplantation. Front Med, 2019, 13 (3): 354-364.

[21] KHOURY HJ, CORTES J, BACCARANI M, et al. Omacetaxine mepesuccinate in patients with advanced chronic myeloid leukemia with resistance or intolerance to tyrosine kinase inhibitors. Leuk Lymphoma, 2015, 56 (1): 120-127.

[22] TANG X, SONG YH, SUN A, et al. Successful treatment of relapsed acute myeloid leukemia without chemotherapy. J Clin Oncol, 2016, 34 (13): e117-e119.

[23] PRZESPOLEWSKI A, SZELES A, WANG ES. Advances in immunotherapy for acute myeloid leukemia. Future Oncol, 2018, 14 (10): 963-978.

[24] CUI Q, QIAN C, XU N, et al. CD38-directed CAR-T cell therapy: A novel immunotherapy strategy for relapsed acute myeloid leukemia after allogeneic hematopoietic stem cell transplantation. J Hematol Oncol, 2021, 14 (1): 82.

[25] QU C, LI Z, KANG L, et al. Successful treatment of two relapsed/refractory t (8; 21) acute myeloid leukemia patients by CD19-directed chimeric antigen receptor T cells. Bone Marrow Transplant, 2019, 54 (7): 1138-1140.

[26] MA YJ, DAI HP, CUI QY, et al. Successful application of PD-1 knockdown CLL1 CAR-T therapy in two AML patients with post-transplant relapse and failure of anti-CD38 CAR-T cell treatment. Am J Cancer Res, 2022, 12 (2): 615-621.

[27] LEOTTA S, CONDORELLI A, SCIORTINO R, et al. Prevention and treatment of acute myeloid leukemia relapse after hematopoietic stem cell transplantation: The state of the art and future perspectives. J Clin Med, 2022, 11 (1): 253.

[28] ZHANG C, WANG XQ, ZHANG RL, et al. Donor-derived CD19 CAR-T cell therapy of relapse of CD19-positive B-ALL post allotransplant. Leukemia, 2021, 35 (6): 1563-1570.

[29] WANG N, HU X, CAO W, et al. Efficacy and safety of CAR19/22 T-cell cocktail therapy in patients with refractory/relapsed B-cell malignancies. Blood, 2020, 135 (1): 17-27.

[30] NCCN Guidelines Version 1. 2021 Acute Lymphoblastic Leukemia.

[31] PAN J, TAN Y, WANG G, et al. Donor-derived CD7 chimeric antigen receptor T cells for T-cell acute lymphoblastic leukemia: First-in-human, phase I trial. J Clin Oncol, 2021, 39 (30): 3340-3351.

[32] KANTARJIAN HM, DEANGELO DJ, STELLJES M, et al. Inotuzumab ozogamicin versus standard therapy for acute lymphoblastic leukemia. N Engl J Med, 2016, 375 (8): 740-753.

[33] 史殷雪, 张晓辉, 许兰平, 等. 化疗联合供者淋巴细胞输注对异基因造血干细胞移植后微小残留病阳性患者慢性移植物抗宿主病及预后的影响. 中华血液学杂志, 2019, 40 (9): 713-719.

[34] KAYSER S, SARTOR C, LUSKIN MR, et al. Outcome of relapsed or refractory acute B-lymphoblastic leukemia patients and BCR-ABL-positive blast cell crisis of B-lymphoid lineage with extramedullary disease receiving inotuzumab ozogamicin. Haematologica, 2022, 107 (9): 2064-2071.

[35] NISHIMOTO M, NAKAMAE H, KOH KR, et al. Dasatinib maintenance therapy after allogeneic hematopoietic stem cell transplantation for an isolated central nervous system blast crisis in chronic myelogenous leukemia. Acta Haematol, 2013, 130 (2): 111-114.

11 异基因造血干细胞移植后随访

移植时间	I 级推荐	II 级推荐	III 级推荐
出院至 +100 天	**频率**：+1 个月内每周评估，+1 个月后隔周直至 +2 个月，之后每月评估或直至出现症状 **内容**：①全面体检，重点关注有无 aGVHD、感染和肺部合并症表现，血常规、肝肾功能、免疫抑制剂浓度、CMV-DNA、EBV-DNA；②+1 个月评估嵌合率；③定期评估原发病		
+3 个月之后	**频率**：+1 年内每月评估或直至出现症状 **内容**：①全面体检，关注有无 GVHD 的表现；②血常规、生化全项、免疫抑制剂浓度；③定期评估原发病；④定期评估嵌合体（AA 患者）；⑤ 17 岁以下患者每 3 个月测量身高、体重		
长期	**频率**：取决于随访期间的症状，若无症状每 6 个月评估至 +3 年，之后每年评估 **内容**：①全面体检，包括妇科和内分泌系统；②定期评估原发病；③定期评估嵌合率（AA 患者）；④定期评估第二肿瘤		

【注释】

随着 HSCT 患者移植后存活时间延长,晚期效应成为影响患者健康状态的重要因素。晚期效应一般指移植后存活半年以上患者出现的各种器官的慢性并发症,移植后长期随访需关注晚期效应,以改善患者健康状态和生存质量[1-5]。

特异性器官长期随访评估表见附录19。

参考文献

[1] DEFILIPP Z, DUARTE RF, SNOWDEN JA, et al. Metabolic syndrome and cardiovascular disease after hematopoietic cell transplantation: Screening and preventive practice recommendations from the cibmtr and ebmT. Biol Blood Marrow Transplant, 2016, 22 (8): 1493-1503.

[2] DIETZ AC, MEHTA PA, VLACHOS A, et al. Current knowledge and priorities for future research in late effects after hematopoietic cell transplantation for inherited bone marrow failure syndromes: Consensus statement from the second pediatric blood and marrow transplant consortium international conference on late effects after pediatric hematopoietic cell transplantation. Biol Blood Marrow Transplant, 2017, 23 (5): 726-735.

[3] MO XD, XU LP, LIU DH, et al. Patients receiving HLA-haploidentical/partially matched related allo-HSCT can achieve desirable health-related QoL that is comparable to that of patients receiving HLA-identical sibling allo-HSCT. Bone Marrow Transplant, 2012, 47 (9): 1201-1205.

[4] DYER G, GILROY N, BRADFORD J, et al. A survey of fertility and sexual health following allogeneic haematopoietic stem cell transplantation in New South Wales, Australia. Br J Haematol, 2016, 172 (4): 592-601.

[5] MO XD, XU LP, LIU DH, et al. Nonmalignant late effects in survivors of partially matched donor hematopoietic stem cell transplantation. Biol Blood Marrow Transplant, 2013, 19 (5): 777-783.

自体造血干细胞移植

1 适应证

1.1 淋巴瘤自体移植适应证

	I级推荐	II级推荐	III级推荐
B细胞淋巴瘤	初始治疗巩固移植： 套细胞淋巴瘤； 高危弥漫大B细胞淋巴瘤（IPI评分3~5分或aaIPI评分2~3分）； 原发或继发中枢神经系统侵袭性淋巴瘤	初始治疗巩固移植： 高级别B细胞淋巴瘤，双打击； 高级别B细胞淋巴瘤，非特指型； 一线治疗强度欠充分的高危伯基特淋巴瘤	初始治疗巩固移植： 进展期（超腔）原发纵隔大B细胞淋巴瘤
	复发/难治后挽救移植： 挽救治疗敏感的复发/难治弥漫大B细胞淋巴瘤； 一线治疗后24个月内复发且二线治疗敏感，或多线治疗敏感的滤泡淋巴瘤； 挽救治疗敏感的伴有大细胞转化的滤泡淋巴瘤/边缘带细胞淋巴瘤； 挽救治疗敏感的套细胞淋巴瘤（一线未接受auto-HSCT）	复发/难治后挽救移植： 挽救治疗敏感的伯基特淋巴瘤	

淋巴瘤自体移植适应证(续)

	I 级推荐	II 级推荐	III 级推荐
NK/T细胞淋巴瘤	初始治疗巩固移植: 侵袭性外周T细胞淋巴瘤(除外局限期可放疗的NK/T细胞淋巴瘤、成年人T细胞淋巴瘤白血病、肝脾γδT细胞淋巴瘤、低危间ALK+间变大T细胞淋巴瘤); 淋巴母细胞淋巴瘤	初始治疗巩固移植: 肝脾γδT细胞淋巴瘤; 进展期NK/T细胞淋巴瘤或局限期原发鼻外且不能行放疗的NK/T细胞淋巴瘤	
		复发/难治后挽救移植: 挽救治疗敏感且不能接受异基因造血干细胞移植的侵袭性T细胞淋巴瘤; 挽救治疗敏感且不能接受异基因造血干细胞移植的淋巴母细胞淋巴瘤	
霍奇金淋巴瘤	挽救治疗敏感的复发/难治霍奇金淋巴瘤		

【注释】

利妥昔单抗时代研究提示，年轻初治套细胞淋巴瘤一线治疗达到完全缓解者行 auto-HSCT 巩固治疗可改善 PFS，其 OS 获益差异无统计学意义[1]。对于初治弥漫大 B 细胞淋巴瘤一线治疗达到完全缓解的患者，SWOG 9704 研究提示，IPI 评分为 3~5 分患者一线巩固 auto-HSCT 后，2 年 PFS 率较未移植患者提高 13%（69% vs. 56%），两组 OS 差异无统计学意义；但 IPI 评分为 4~5 分患者 auto-HSCT 后 2 年 OS 率为 82%，显著优于未移植组（2 年 OS 率 64%，$P=0.01$）[2]。DLCL04 研究提示，auto-HSCT 可延长 aaIPI 评分为 2~3 分患者的 PFS 时间[3]。我国一项多中心回顾性临床研究提示，对于中期疗效评价达到部分缓解或完全缓解的中高危弥漫大 B 细胞淋巴瘤患者，行 auto-HSCT 可显著改善 OS 及 PFS[4]。

在高级别 B 细胞淋巴瘤双打击亚型中，auto-HSCT 的一线巩固治疗地位仍有争议，有研究证实在一线治疗强度不足时（如 R-CHOP 方案），联合 auto-HSCT 组较未移植组复发时间推迟，但当一线治疗强度充足时（如 DA-EPOCH-R、R-hyper-CVAD、R-CODOX-M/IVAC 等方案），行 auto-HSCT 未见显著获益[5]。对于高级别 B 细胞淋巴瘤，非特指型或双表达大 B 细胞淋巴瘤，目前尚未有充分的研究证实可从 auto-HSCT 中获益。但考虑到高级别 B 细胞淋巴瘤，非特指型患者预后不佳，美国国立综合癌症网络（NCCN）指南建议部分中心可尝试对该类型患者行 auto-HSCT 巩固治疗。

原发中枢弥漫大 B 细胞淋巴瘤多项随机对照研究探索全脑放疗及 auto-HSCT 两种巩固治疗方案的有效性，结果显示两种巩固治疗有效性相似，全脑放疗以远期认知功能受损为主要不良反应，auto-HSCT 以血液学不良反应为主要不良反应[6-7]。考虑到全脑放疗对患者远期生命质量的影响，本工作组推荐对于一线治疗有效且能耐受 auto-HSCT 的原发中枢弥漫大 B 细胞淋巴瘤患者行 auto-HSCT 巩固治疗。对于原发纵隔大 B 细胞淋巴瘤，目前尚鲜见研究探索 auto-HSCT 巩固治疗的价值，考虑到进展期原发纵隔大 B 细胞淋巴瘤预后不佳（主要是淋巴瘤侵及横膈以下），且进入复发/难治状态挽救治疗有效率显著低于弥漫大 B 细胞淋巴瘤者[8]，故可考虑一线接受 auto-HSCT 巩固治疗。伯基特淋巴瘤是高侵袭性淋巴瘤，标准治疗为采用强化疗方案（如 Hyper-CVAD、CODOX-M、DA-EOPCH）以求达到治愈，而一旦进入复发/难治状态则疾病可快速进展、危及生命，当一线治疗有效但是治疗强度不足（化疗减量或化疗延迟）时，参照高级别 B 细胞双打击淋巴瘤的研究经验，可考虑接受 auto-HSCT 巩固治疗以增加治疗强度。

侵袭性外周 T 细胞淋巴瘤是一组高度异质性疾病，涵盖多个病理亚型，除 ALK+ 间变大 T 细胞淋巴瘤亚型外，其余亚型均预后不良，目前虽缺乏大样本量前瞻性随机对照研究证实 auto-HSCT 在一线巩固治疗中的地位，但单臂研究或前瞻性对照研究均提示 auto-HSCT 可能部分改善患者生存[9-10]。成年人 T 细胞淋巴瘤白血病、肝脾 γδT 细胞淋巴瘤因预后极差，而且侵及骨髓，推荐一旦诱导治疗有效者尽快接受异基因造血干细胞移植。进展期 NK/T 细胞淋巴瘤或局限期原发鼻外且不能进行放疗的 NK/T 细胞淋巴瘤侵袭性强，一线治疗缓解后推荐接受 auto-HSCT，极高危患者可考虑接受异基因造血干细胞移植。而 ALK+ 间变大 T 细胞淋巴瘤因预后较好，不同指南对其接受 auto-HSCT 的指征有争议，推荐采用分层管理，IPI 评分高危者接受 auto-HSCT，而低危者可暂不考虑 auto-HSCT，其余亚型侵袭性外周 T 细胞淋巴瘤一线治疗有效者推荐接受 auto-HSCT 巩固治疗。

淋巴母细胞淋巴瘤起源于较成熟 B/T 细胞更早的前体淋巴细胞阶段，具有部分白血病特征，对诱导治疗达到首次缓解的淋巴母细胞淋巴瘤患者，行 auto-HSCT 或异基因造血干细胞移植巩固治疗均可改善患者 PFS，但 OS 的改善差异无统计学意义[11-13]。auto-HSCT 与异基因造血干细胞移植相比，OS

时间差异亦无统计学意义[14]。但 auto-HSCT 存在复发率高的缺点，同时考虑到异基因造血干细胞移植的治疗相关死亡率高、经济负担及对生命质量的影响，双次 auto-HSCT 可能是淋巴母细胞淋巴瘤患者新的选择。一项我国自主发起的前瞻性对照多中心临床研究结果显示，双次 auto-HSCT 可最大限度清除患者肿瘤细胞，减少复发，与异基因造血干细胞移植相比，具有安全性高、移植相关死亡率低的优点。双次、单次 auto-HSCT 患者的 3 年复发率分别为 36.5%、53.1%，双次 auto-HSCT 患者的 3 年无病生存（DFS）率及 OS 率分别为 73.5%、76.3%，显著优于单次 auto-HSCT 组。年轻（<32 岁）患者及第 1 次移植后达到完全缓解患者将更有好的生存获益[15]。对于初始骨髓侵犯比例不高且经诱导治疗快速达到全身及骨髓缓解的淋巴母细胞淋巴瘤患者，推荐行 auto-HSCT 巩固治疗。

1.2 多发性骨髓瘤自体造血干细胞移植适应证

	I 级推荐	II 级推荐	III 级推荐
年龄	ASCT 的最适宜年龄是 ≤65 岁	对于体质好,没有明显器官功能不全的患者,ASCT 的年龄延长至 70 岁	
心功能	美国纽约心脏病学会(NYHA)心功能分级 ≤2 级		
活动状态	ECOG 活动状态评分 ≤2 分		
肾功能	血 Cr ≥ 60ml/min 血 30ml/min ≤ Cr<60ml/min,尿量正常,应将预处理剂量减量 血 Cr<30ml/min,应权衡移植的利弊		
血压	收缩压 ≥ 90mmHg		
肝功能	胆红素 <2mg/dl		
血氧饱和度	静息状态下 SpO_2>95%		
乙肝病毒	乙肝大三阳或 HBV-DNA 超过正常值——不适合移植		
其他	患者不能有心理疾患		

注：年龄：欧洲将 ASCT 年龄限制为 70~75 岁。在我国，如果年龄<70 岁，GA 评分为 FIT 的患者，也可以接受 ASCT。

心功能：是指移植前评估的心功能，而不是诱导治疗前的心功能。

肾功能不全：血肌酐>300μmol/L 的 MM 患者不建议 ASCT，但是如果有血液替代治疗条件的 MM 患者可以接受 ASCT 的报道。此类患者行 ASCT 副作用明显增加，移植相关死亡率达到 15%。

肝功能：如果患者为乙肝携带者（乙肝小三阳且 HBV-DNA–）在预防抗乙肝病毒基础上可以接受 ASCT；如果患者为乙肝携带者在诱导治疗期间间断出现 HBV-DNA+，不建议移植；有肝硬化或者肝脏淀粉样变性，不建议接受 ASCT。

肺功能：如果患者有慢性肺间质性疾病不建议接受 ASCT。

2 动员方案

2.1 干细胞动员方案与冻存

2.1.1 干细胞动员方案

Ⅰ类推荐	Ⅱ类推荐
依托泊苷 +G-CSF（1 类）	G-CSF（2 类）
环磷酰胺 +G-CSF（1A 类）	环磷酰胺 +G-CSF+ 普乐沙福（2 类）
G-CSF+ 普乐沙福（1 类）	E-CHOP+ G-CSF（2B 类） 疾病特异性化疗 + 粒细胞集落刺激因子（G-CSF）动员

注：对于发病时伴有浆细胞瘤或者外周血循环浆细胞者建议使用化疗动员。

对于既往接受超过 4 疗程、老年、诱导治疗造血恢复慢、使用多种对干细胞采集有影响的药物如（免疫调节剂、亚硝基脲类、烷化剂），建议使用稳态动员。

对于化疗动员效果欠佳，可以在此基础上加用普乐沙福。建议在移植前采集足够二次移植的干细胞量。

可以根据采集前外周血 $CD34^+$ 细胞比例决定是否使用普乐沙福及干细胞采集。

接受单次 ASCT 需要的干细胞量最好 $\geqslant 2 \times 10^6$/kg。

淋巴瘤初治患者一般在化疗 4 个周期后病情缓解（完全缓解或部分缓解）时动员采集造血干细胞。复发/难治患者挽救治疗 2 个周期后，如治疗有效（完全缓解或部分缓解）且骨髓未受到侵犯，应尽早考虑动员并采集造血干细胞。计划移植的患者应尽量避免选择损伤骨髓干细胞的药物，如氟达拉滨、苯达莫司汀、来那度胺等（或造血干细胞采集前来那度胺至少停药 2~4 周）。

2.1.2 干细胞冻存

干细胞冻存需要 –80℃冰箱和液氮。

注：干细胞冻存保护液为白蛋白 + 二甲基亚砜（DMSO）+ 甲基纤维素 +RPMI-1640 培养基。

–80℃冰箱冻存每年损失干细胞 5% 左右。如果是延迟移植需要冻存足够多的干细胞。

液氮冻存每年损失干细胞 1% 左右。

2.2 造血干细胞采集

2.2.1 采集时机

应用 G-CSF 3 天后开始监测外周血 $CD34^+$ 细胞绝对计数，外周血 $CD34^+$ 细胞绝对计数升高至 5~10/μl 以上时可考虑开始采集；若外周血 $CD34^+$ 细胞绝对计数<10/μl 建议联合普乐沙福（0.24mg/kg）。

单平台方法是 $CD34^+$ 细胞绝对计数的首选方法，该方法减少了室间变异和多台仪器间的系统误差。操作中需要注意：严格按照操作说明书调整细胞和抗体的最佳比；推荐采用反向抽吸法加样，以保证加入准确体积的样本和已知浓度的定量荧光微球；为避免荧光微球的丢失，在裂解细胞后不进行离心洗涤。

2.2.2 采集目标值

优质动员目标值为 $CD34^+$ 细胞 $\geqslant 5 \times 10^6/kg$，达标动员目标值为 $CD34^+$ 细胞 $\geqslant 2 \times 10^6/kg$；未达标但 $CD34^+$ 细胞 $\geqslant 1 \times 10^6/kg$（单个核细胞数 $\geqslant 2 \times 10^8/kg$）也可根据患者情况考虑行 auto-HSCT。

2.2.3 采集过程中注意事项

自体造血干细胞采集前需评估患者血管条件，可选择外周静脉（首选肘正中静脉）进行一次性静脉穿刺或选择颈内、股静脉进行双腔导管置管。采集天数通常不超过 3 天，每天采集时间不宜超过 5 小时，以免后面收集到的细胞活性下降。循环血量每次 8 000~12 000ml，也可根据患者体质量适当调节循环血量（一般不超过患者血容量的 3 倍）。适时采用手动收集，手动控制开始收集和终止收集的时间能更准确收集到白膜层。采集过程中，为预防发生低血钙（主要表现为面部、手足、四肢麻木，严重者可出现抽搐或呕吐症状），可给予静脉滴注或口服葡萄糖酸钙注射液。

3 临床应用

3.1 自体造血干细胞移植治疗多发性骨髓瘤

3.1.1 移植前评估

	Ⅰ级推荐	Ⅱ级推荐	Ⅲ级推荐
病史采集和体格检查	完整的病史采集 体格检查 体能状态评估		
实验室检查	血常规，网织红细胞计数，白细胞分类 尿常规，尿沉渣流式分析 24小时尿轻链定量；24小时尿总蛋白及24小时尿白蛋白定量 血清免疫球蛋白定量；血免疫固定电泳 血清蛋白电泳；M蛋白定量 血清游离轻链（FLC）定量 血生化［至少应该包括肝肾功能、血钙、乳酸脱氢酶、碱性磷酸酶；血肌酐及钙；血氨基末端脑钠肽前体（NT-proBNP），心肌肌钙蛋白Ⅰ（cTNI）］	尿固定电泳	

移植前评估(续)

	I 级推荐	II 级推荐	III 级推荐
骨髓穿刺	形态学分析 二代流式/二代测序分析		
其他影像学检查	心电图,心脏、肝、肾超声 肺部高分辨 CT、肺功能 浆细胞瘤评估(如果有)		

注:新诊断时不论是否已做 FISH 及染色体,此时不必复查。

建议使用二代流式及二代测序(检查 IgH 及 IgL V 表达谱)检测 MRD,而不是 NGS 检查是否有基因突变。

不必复查骨病,除非有浆细胞瘤。

如果基线做了 PET-CT,可以复查对比 SUV 值变化。

3.1.2 干细胞移植时机

缓解深度	诱导治疗后获得部分缓解(PR)及以上疗效
移植时机的选择	早移植相比晚移植:两种方案总体疗效相似,但是推荐行早移植

注:早期 ASCT.从诊断到移植 12 个月内;延迟 ASCT:待复发后移植。

复发后行 ASCT 是可行的,但是患者可能在复发后丧失移植时机。因此,早期 ASCT 仍是符合移植条件的初治 MM 患者的标准治疗。

3.1.3 诱导治疗

Ⅰ类推荐	Ⅱ类推荐
硼替佐米+来那度胺+地塞米松（BRD）	硼替佐米+地塞米松（BD）
卡非佐米+来那度胺+地塞米松（KRD）	来那度胺+地塞米松（RD）
硼替佐米+环磷酰胺+地塞米松（BCD）	环磷酰胺+来那度胺+地塞米松（CRD）
卡非佐米+环磷酰胺+地塞米松（KCD）	环磷酰胺+沙利度胺+地塞米松（CTD）
硼替佐米+多柔比星+地塞米松（BAD）	沙利度胺+多柔比星+地塞米松（TAD）
硼替佐米+沙利度胺+地塞米松（BTD）	
伊沙佐米+来那度胺+地塞米松（IRD）	
达雷妥尤单抗+BRD（D-BRD）	
达雷妥尤单抗+BTD（D-BTD）	
达雷妥尤单抗+KRD（D-KRD）	

注：建议使用含蛋白酶体抑制剂、免疫调节剂、单克隆抗体等新药的联合化疗。
以含蛋白酶体抑制剂和免疫调节剂两类新药的方案为首选。
如果伴有浆细胞瘤或者循环浆细胞的患者，建议使用含细胞毒药物的联合治疗。
诱导治疗的疗程数为3~6疗程。
获得PR及以上疗效就可以接受自体干细胞移植，不追求移植前一定获得深度缓解。

3.1.4 预处理

Ⅰ类推荐	Ⅱ类推荐
美法仑 200mg/m²	美法仑 + 马利兰 美法仑 + 苯达莫司汀 马利兰 + 环磷酰胺 +VP16 卡氮芥 +VP16+Ara-C+ 白消安（BEAM）

注：美法仑 200mg/m² 是标准的预处理方案；肌酐清除率<30ml/min 的 ASCT 患者，应将美法仑预处理剂量降为 140mg/m²。

70 岁以上的患者，如果接受 ASCT，也需要根据生理健康评分、合并症和病情的侵袭性进行综合临床判断美法仑使用剂量，美法仑最低剂量为 140mg/m²。

在美法仑的基础上加用其他药物，可能提高疗效，但是不良反应明显增加。

在美法仑基础上加用其他药物适用于伴浆细胞瘤或者发病时有循环浆细胞。

预处理前应该请口腔科、耳鼻喉科、肛肠外科会诊，排查潜在的感染灶。

口服预防细菌、真菌及病毒感染的药物。

3.1.5 双次移植

1. 伴高危细胞遗传学异常、首次 ASCT 后尚未获得 VGPR 及以上疗效的患者，建议在首次 ASCT 后的 6 个月左右进行第二次 ASCT。
2. 首次移植复发后，再诱导治疗缓解后挽救性 ASCT。
3. 预处理：美法仑 $200mg/m^2$。

【注释】

序贯二次移植：第一次移植后间隔 6 个月左右进行的二次移植。

挽救性二次移植：复发后再诱导缓解后进行的移植。

非清髓或者清髓性异基因移植建议用于序贯二次移植或者挽救性二次移植。

3.1.6 巩固治疗

1. 干细胞移植后 3 个月左右进行。
2. 适用于移植后没有获得 VGPR 或 CR 患者。
3. 与诱导治疗药物、治疗强度相似的方案。
4. 2~4 疗程，根据患者耐受性决定疗程数。

3.1.7 维持治疗

Ⅰ级推荐	Ⅱ级推荐	Ⅲ级推荐
来那度胺 伊沙佐米 硼替佐米	沙利度胺 来那度胺 + 硼替佐米 来那度胺 + 伊沙佐米 达雷妥尤单抗 来那度胺 + 卡非佐米	来那度胺 + 达雷妥尤单抗 泊马度胺

【注释】

1. 细胞遗传学标危患者可用单药维持治疗。
2. 细胞遗传学高危患者,建议使用两药联合(免疫调节剂 + 蛋白酶体抑制剂或单抗)维持治疗。
3. 细胞遗传学标危患者可能从二药维持治疗中获益更多。
4. 维持治疗 2 年或更长时间。
5. 维持治疗是否加用激素根据患者耐受性决定。
6. 泊马度胺可以作为诱导治疗后的序贯治疗(维持治疗)。

3.1.8 随访复查

1. 每 3 个月一次的检查
（1）血常规、生化、肝肾功能、免疫球蛋白定量及固定电泳 M 蛋白定量；血清游离轻链定量。
（2）尿常规、24 小时尿总蛋白、白蛋白及 24 小时尿轻链定量。
2. MRD 检查　二代流式或二代测序任选。
3. 骨病或浆细胞瘤　根据需要检测，不做常规要求。
4. 骨髓穿刺　根据需要检测，不做常规要求。

3.2 自体造血干细胞移植治疗淋巴瘤

3.2.1 auto-HSCT 预处理

常用预处理方案参考剂量 *

BEAM 方案			
卡莫司汀	300mg/m²	i.v.	第 -7 天
依托泊苷	200mg/m²	i.v.	第 -6~-3 天
阿糖胞苷	200mg/m²	i.v.	第 -6~-3 天
美法仑	140mg/m²	i.v.	第 -2 天

*. 各中心可根据实际情况酌情调整。

BEAC 方案			
卡莫司汀	300mg/m²	i.v.	第 -7 天
依托泊苷	200mg/m²	i.v.	第 -6~-3 天
阿糖胞苷	200mg/m²	i.v.	第 -6~-3 天
环磷酰胺	1g/m²	i.v.	第 -6~-3 天
CBV 方案			
卡莫司汀	300mg/m²	i.v.	第 -6 天
依托泊苷	200mg/m²	i.v.	第 -5~-2 天
环磷酰胺	1.2~1.8g/m²	i.v.	第 -5~-2 天
TBI/Cy 方案			
TBI	10~12Gy（总照射剂量）		第 -6~-4 天
环磷酰胺	60mg/kg	i.v.	第 -3~-2 天

注：TBI 推荐分次照射，2~3 次均可，如果条件不允许也可以单次照射，但总剂量不宜超过 8Gy。

BCNU+TT 方案			
卡莫司汀	400mg/m²	i.v.	第 -6 天
塞替派	5mg/kg q12h	i.v.	第 -5~-4 天

TEAM 方案			
塞替派	8mg/kg	i.v.	第 -7 天
依托泊苷	200mg/m²	i.v.	第 -6~-3 天
阿糖胞苷	200mg/m²	i.v.	第 -6~-3 天
美法仑	140mg/m²	i.v.	第 -2 天

注：对于既往伴有或出现肺部问题的患者也可考虑用塞替派代替卡莫司汀，以避免卡莫司汀导致的肺部不良反应。

BeEAM 方案			
苯达莫司汀	120~180mg/m²	i.v.	第 -8~-7 天
依托泊苷	200mg/m²	i.v.	第 -6~-3 天
阿糖胞苷	200mg/m²	i.v.	第 -6~-3 天
美法仑	140mg/m²	i.v.	第 -2 天

SEAM 方案			
司莫司汀	250mg/m²	i.v.	第 –7 天
依托泊苷	200mg/m²	i.v.	第 –6~–3 天
阿糖胞苷	200mg/m²	i.v.	第 –6~–3 天
美法仑	140mg/m²	i.v.	第 –2 天

【注释】

淋巴瘤 auto-HSCT 前预处理指在造血干细胞回输前对患者进行大剂量化疗和/或放疗，旨在进一步清除体内肿瘤细胞，并为干细胞植入创造条件。

目前常用的预处理方案分为单纯化疗方案及以全身照射（TBI）为基础的放化疗联合预处理方案，预处理方案的选择主要取决于各中心经验。常用单纯化疗方案包括 BEAM（卡莫司汀、依托泊苷、阿糖胞苷、美法仑）[24] 和 CBV（环磷酰胺、卡莫司汀、依托泊苷）[25]，以及由其衍生的 BEAC（将 BEAM 方案中美法仑替换为环磷酰胺）[26]；在卡莫司汀无法获得情况下可将其替换，如 TEAM（将 BEAM 方案中卡莫司汀替换为塞替派）[27]、BeEAM（将 BEAM 方案中卡莫司汀替换为苯达莫司汀）[28-29]、SEAM/LEAM（将 BEAM 方案中卡莫司汀替换为司莫司汀、福莫司汀或洛莫司汀）[30-31] 等。此外，Bu/Cy（白消安、环磷酰胺）方案、GBM（吉西他滨、白消安、美法仑）方案等也越来越受到重视[32]。

原发中枢神经系统淋巴瘤建议选择以塞替派为基础的预处理方案，如卡莫司汀联合塞替派（BCNU+TT），白消安、环磷酰胺联合塞替派（TBC），可提高auto-HSCT疗效，且耐受性良好[6, 33]。

含TBI的预处理方案中常用TBI总剂量为10~12Gy，分次放疗。常联合其他化疗药物如大剂量环磷酰胺，但以TBI为基础的预处理方案患者第二肿瘤（尤其是骨髓增生异常综合征/急性髓系白血病）发生明显增加，且部分患者计划或已接受达到器官受照限量的局部放疗剂量，因而制约了TBI的应用[34-37]。

3.2.2 auto-HSCT相关并发症及处理原则

接受auto-HSCT的患者可发生多种并发症，包括中性粒细胞减少、肺部并发症、出血及血栓相关并发症、黏膜炎、腹泻、第二肿瘤等。现对于常见并发症的处理简述如下。

1. 中性粒细胞减少伴发热　很常见，主要原因为革兰氏阴性杆菌引起的血行感染，需要通过血培养等病原学检查帮助诊断，对于高危粒细胞缺乏患者可预防性使用氟喹诺酮类药物，一线经验性抗感染治疗应选择能覆盖铜绿假单胞菌和其他严重革兰氏阴性杆菌的广谱抗菌药物，在某些特定情况下需要同时覆盖严重的革兰氏阳性球菌（具体参照《中国中性粒细胞缺乏伴发热患者抗菌药物临床应用指南》）。在抗菌药物治疗无效时，需考虑真菌、病毒和其他病原菌感染，参照相关指南和共识尽早开始抗真菌和其他病原菌的治疗。增加移植前1~2周肠道净化的处理。

2. 肺部并发症　主要为感染性和非感染性。非感染性肺损伤主要包括肺水肿、特发性肺炎（IPS）、放化疗相关肺损伤等。IPS可由多种病因共同导致，包括弥漫性肺泡出血（DAH）、围植入期呼吸窘迫综合征等。间质性肺损伤常见于造血重建过程中,如出现不明原因发热需及时通过行胸部 CT 平扫、完善病原学检查等进行鉴别,对于非感染性的间质性肺损伤通常需要激素治疗及吸氧、控制液体平衡等支持治疗。

3. 出血并发症　最常见的原因是血小板减少。肠道、肺或中枢神经系统等部位出血可以是致命性的。辐照血小板输注、抗纤溶药物等为预防出血并发症的常见治疗方式,尚没有资料显示白细胞介素 11 和重组人促血小板生成素在预防出血方面有积极作用。

4. 血栓并发症　主要包括深静脉血栓栓塞、导管相关血栓形成等,需要根据血小板计数、有无活动性出血、肾小球滤过率等评估是否进行抗凝治疗。进行治疗选择时需要综合考虑出血和血栓并发症的风险权衡利弊。

5. 黏膜炎　通常出现在移植极期,处理多以抗感染、局部消毒、镇痛及补充维生素等为主要手段,如果未发展为严重感染,多在中性粒细胞恢复后缓解。

3.2.3 auto-HSCT 患者的护理

1. 病房环境准备　百级层流洁净病房或达标的简易层流设备,每月进行空气、物表、手部卫生等微生物监测;每日按照移植病房全环境保护要求清洁消毒病房;层流病房内所有物品需清洁消毒后使用;医护人员进入层流病房前严格执行手部卫生规范。

2. 移植患者护理常规　对患者既往健康情况、易感部位、症状、风险、导管、心理进行全面评估;入层流病房后给予特级护理及心电监护,详细做好各项护理记录;实施保护性隔离措施,严格遵守各项无菌操作规程；每日观察中心静脉导管及易感部位情况，密切监测患者生命体征及用药后反应，准确记录出入量。

3. 预防感染护理　患者注意手卫生，避免感染；给予滴眼液滴眼睛、药物涂鼻腔 3 次 /d；保持皮肤清洁，观察口腔黏膜情况，用软毛牙刷刷牙，漱口液漱口 4~6 次 /d。预处理化疗后，口腔护理 2 次 /d；观察肛门周围黏膜情况，坐浴 2 次 /d。

4. 自体造血干细胞回输护理　自体造血干细胞由专人复苏及回输，严格执行双人核对制度；准备符合要求的输注通路，必须取下输液接头，干细胞现复苏、现输注，注意生命体征变化及患者的不适主诉；收集干细胞做细菌培养并将储血袋按照医疗垃圾处理。

5. 饮食原则　患者饮食需微波炉高火加热 5 分钟进行消毒，禁止吃剩饭菜；移植患者饮食应清淡，采用新鲜食材，制作过程干净卫生，忌生冷辛辣及海鲜，应少油、少渣易消化、少刺激性的饮食，避免食用带刺、含骨头等坚硬的食物；口服药物后，进餐应与服药时间有间隔，避免呕吐。

6. 心理护理　提供舒适、安静、清洁、整齐的病房环境，和患者协商制订良好的作息时间；与患者建立相互信赖的关系，鼓励患者倾诉，排除患者紧张焦虑的因素，引导患者正确对待疾病，增强治愈疾病的信心。家属积极配合，探视时提供正能量，给予患者良好的心理支持。

参考文献

[1] GERSON JN, HANDORF E, VILLA D, et al. Survival outcomes of younger patients with mantle cell lymphoma treated in the rituximab era. J Clin Oncol, 2019, 37 (6): 471-480.

[2] STIFF PJ, UNGER JM, COOK JR, et al. Autologous transplantation as consolidation for aggressive non-Hodgkin's lymphoma. N Engl J Med, 2013, 369 (18): 1681-1690.

[3] CHIAPPELLA A, MARTELLI M, ANGELUCCI E, et al. Rituximab-dose-dense chemotherapy with or without high-dose chemotherapy plus autologous stem-cell transplantation in high-risk diffuse large B-cell lymphoma (DLCL04): Final results of a multicentre, open-label, randomised, controlled, phase 3 study. Lancet Oncol, 2017, 18 (8): 1076-1088.

[4] WEN Q, GAO L, XIONG JK, et al. High-dose chemotherapy combined with autologous hematopoietic stem cell transplantation as frontline therapy for intermediate/high-risk diffuse large B cell lymphoma. Curr Med Sci, 2021, 41 (3): 465-473.

[5] LANDSBURG DJ, FALKIEWICZ MK, MALY J, et al. Outcomes of patients with double-hit lymphoma who achieve first complete remission. J Clin Oncol, 2017, 35 (20): 2260-2267.

[6] FERRERI AJ, ILLERHAUS G. The role of autologous stem cell transplantation in primary central nervous system lymphoma. Blood, 2016, 127 (13): 1642-1649.

[7] HOUILLIER C, TAILLANDIER L, DUREAU S, et al. Radiotherapy or autologous stem-cell transplantation for primary CNS lymphoma in patients 60 years of age and younger: Results of the Intergroup ANOCEF-GOELAMS Randomized Phase II PRECIS Study. J Clin Oncol, 2019, 37 (10): 823-833.

[8] KURUVILLA J, PINTILIE M, TSANG R, et al. Salvage chemotherapy and autologous stem cell transplantation are inferior for relapsed or refractory primary mediastinal large B-cell lymphoma compared with diffuse large B-cell lymphoma. Leuk Lymphoma, 2008, 49 (7): 1329-1336.

[9] D'AMORE F, RELANDER T, LAURITZSEN GF, et al. Up-front autologous stem-cell transplantation in peripheral T-cell lymphoma: NLG-T-01. J Clin Oncol, 2012, 30 (25): 3093-3099.

[10] PARK SI, HORWITZ SM, FOSS FM, et al. The role of autologous stem cell transplantation in patients with nodal

peripheral T-cell lymphomas in first complete remission: Report from COMPLETE, a prospective, multicenter cohort study. Cancer, 2019, 125 (9): 1507-1517.

[11] SWEETENHAM JW, SANTINI G, QIAN W, et al. High-dose therapy and autologous stem-cell transplantation versus conventional-dose consolidation/maintenance therapy as postremission therapy for adult patients with lymphoblastic lymphoma: Results of a randomized trial of the European Group for Blood and Marrow Transplantation and the United Kingdom Lymphoma Group. J Clin Oncol, 2001, 19 (11): 2927-2936.

[12] YANG L, TAN Y, SHI J, et al. Allogeneic hematopoietic stem cell transplantation should be in preference to conventional chemotherapy as post-remission treatment for adults with lymphoblastic lymphoma. Bone Marrow Transplant, 2018, 53 (10): 1340-1344.

[13] JEONG SH, MOON JH, KIM JS, et al. Multicenter analysis of treatment outcomes in adult patients with lymphoblastic lymphoma who received hyper-CVAD induction followed by hematopoietic stem cell transplantation. Ann Hematol, 2015, 94 (4): 617-625.

[14] LEVINE JE, HARRIS RE, LOBERIZA FR Jr, et al. A comparison of allogeneic and autologous bone marrow transplantation for lymphoblastic lymphoma. Blood, 2003, 101 (7): 2476-2482.

[15] LIU Y, RAO J, LI J, et al. Tandem autologous hematopoietic stem cell transplantation for treatment of adult T-cell lymphoblastic lymphoma: A multiple center prospective study in China. Haematologica, 2021, 106 (1): 163-172.

[16] LINCH DC, WINFIELD D, GOLDSTONE AH, et al. Dose intensification with autologous bone-marrow transplantation in relapsed and resistant Hodgkin's disease: Results of a BNLI randomised trial. Lancet, 1993, 341 (8852): 1051-1054.

[17] FILETTI S, DURANTE C, HARTL D, et al. Thyroid cancer: ESMO clinical practice guidelines for diagnosis, treatment and follow-up. Ann Oncol, 2019, 30 (12): 1856-1883.

[18] DHAKAL B, SZABO A, CHHABRA S, et al. Autologous transplantation for newly diagnosed multiple myeloma in

the era of novel agent induction: A systematic review and meta-analysis. JAMA Oncol, 2018, 4 (3): 343-350.
［19］CAVO M. Double vs single autologous stem cell transplantation for newly diagnosed multiple myeloma: Long-term follow-up (10 years) analysis of randomized phase 3 studies. Blood, 2018, 132: 12.
［20］GONSALVES WI, BUADI FK, AILAWADHI S, et al. Utilization of hematopoietic stem cell transplantation for the treatment of multiple myeloma: A Mayo Stratification of Myeloma and Risk-Adapted Therapy (mSMART) consensus statement. Bone Marrow Transplant, 2019, 54 (3): 353-367.
［21］SONNEVELD P, BEKSAC M, VAN DER HOLT B, et al. Consolidation followed by maintenance therapy versus maintenance alone in newly diagnosed, transplant eligible patients with multiple myeloma (MM): A randomized phase 3 study of the European Myeloma Network (EMN02/HO95 MM Trial). Blood, 2016, 128: 242.
［22］中国医药教育协会血液学专业委员会, 中国中西医结合学会血液学专业委员会骨髓瘤专家委员会. 多发性骨髓瘤中西医结合诊疗专家共识 (2019). 中华医学杂志, 2019, 99 (28): 2169-2175.
［23］陈文明. 造血干细胞移植用于多发性骨髓瘤的治疗. 中国实用内科杂志, 2022; 42 (4): 330-335.
［24］MILLS W, CHOPRA R, MCMILLAN A, et al. BEAM chemotherapy and autologous bone marrow transplantation for patients with relapsed or refractory non-Hodgkin's lymphoma. J Clin Oncol, 1995, 13 (3): 588-595.
［25］WEAVER CH, APPELBAUM FR, PETERSEN FB, et al. High-dose cyclophosphamide, carmustine, and etoposide followed by autologous bone marrow transplantation in patients with lymphoid malignancies who have received dose-limiting radiation therapy. J Clin Oncol, 1993, 11 (7): 1329-1335.
［26］ROBINSON SP, BOUMENDIL A, FINEL H, et al. High-dose therapy with BEAC conditioning compared to BEAM conditioning prior to autologous stem cell transplantation for non-Hodgkin lymphoma: No differences in toxicity or outcome. A matched-control study of the EBMT-Lymphoma Working Party. Bone Marrow Transplant, 2018, 53 (12): 1553-1559.
［27］SELLNER L, BOUMENDIL A, FINEL H, et al. Thiotepa-based high-dose therapy for autologous stem cell trans-

plantation in lymphoma: a retrospective study from the EBMT. Bone Marrow Transplant, 2016, 51 (2): 212-218.

[28] VISANI G, STEFANI PM, CAPRIA S, et al. Bendamustine, etoposide, cytarabine, melphalan, and autologous stem cell rescue produce a 72% 3-year PFS in resistant lymphoma. Blood, 2014, 124 (19): 3029-3031.

[29] CHANTEPIE SP, GARCIAZ S, TCHERNONOG E, et al. Bendamustine-based conditioning prior to autologous stem cell transplantation (ASCT): Results of a French multicenter study of 474 patients from LYmphoma Study Association (LYSA) centers. Am J Hematol, 2018, 93 (6): 729-735.

[30] COLITA A, COLITA A, BUMBEA H, et al. LEAM vs. BEAM vs. CLV conditioning regimen for autologous stem cell transplantation in malignant lymphomas: Retrospective comparison of toxicity and efficacy on 222 patients in the first 100 days after transplant, on behalf of the Romanian Society for Bone Marrow Transplantation. Front Oncol, 2019, 9: 892.

[31] OLIVIERI J, MOSNA F, PELOSINI M, et al. A comparison of the conditioning regimens beam and feam for autologous hematopoietic stem cell transplantation in lymphoma: An observational study on 1038 patients from fondazione italiana linfomi. Biol Blood Marrow Transplant, 2018, 24 (9): 1814-1822.

[32] NIETO Y, THALL PF, MA J, et al. Phase Ⅱ trial of high-dose gemcitabine/busulfan/melphalan with autologous stem cell transplantation for primary refractory or poor-risk relapsed Hodgkin lymphoma. Biol Blood Marrow Transplant, 2018, 24 (8): 1602-1609.

[33] OMURO A, CORREA DD, DEANGELIS LM, et al. R-MPV followed by high-dose chemotherapy with TBC and autologous stem-cell transplant for newly diagnosed primary CNS lymphoma. Blood, 2015, 125 (9): 1403-1410.

[34] ILLERHAUS G, MARKS R, IHORST G, et al. High-dose chemotherapy with autologous stem-cell transplantation and hyperfractionated radiotherapy as first-line treatment of primary CNS lymphoma. J Clin Oncol, 2006, 24 (24): 3865-3870.

[35] HOSING C, MUNSELL M, YAZJI S, et al. Risk of therapy-related myelodysplastic syndrome/acute leukemia

following high-dose therapy and autologous bone marrow transplantation for non-Hodgkin's lymphoma. Ann Oncol, 2002, 13 (3): 450-459.

[36] MILLIGAN DW, RUIZ DE ELVIRA MC, KOLB HJ, et al. Secondary leukaemia and myelodysplasia after autografting for lymphoma: Results from the EBMT. EBMT lymphoma and late effects working parties: European group for blood and marrow transplantation. Br J Haematol, 1999, 106 (4): 1020-1026.

[37] DARRINGTON DL, VOSE JM, ANDERSON JR, et al. Incidence and characterization of secondary myelodysplastic syndrome and acute myelogenous leukemia following high-dose chemoradiotherapy and autologous stem-cell transplantation for lymphoid malignancies. J Clin Oncol, 1994, 12 (12): 2527-2534.

附录

附录 1 AML（非 APL）危险分层标准[*]

危险分层	遗传学异常
预后好	t（8；21）（q22；q22.1）；*RUNX1-RUNX1T1* inv（16）（p13.1q22）or t（16；16）（p13.1；q22）；*CBFB-MYH11* Biallelic mutated *CEBPA* Mutated *NPM1* without *FLT3-ITD* or with *FLT3-ITD*^{low}
预后中等	Mutated *NPM1* and *FLT3-ITD*^{high} Wild-type *NPM1* without *FLT3-ITD* or with *FLT3-ITD*^{low}（without adverse-risk genetic lesions） t（9；11）（p21.3；q23.3）；*MLLT3-KMT2A* Cytogenetic abnormalities not classified as favorable or adverse
预后差	t（6；9）（p23；q34.1）；*DEK-NUP214* t（v；11q23.3）；*KMT2A* rearranged t（9；22）（q34.1；q11.2）；*BCR-ABL1* inv（3）（q21.3q26.2）or t（3；3）（q21.3；q26.2）；*GATA2*，*MECOM*（*EVI1*） −5 or del（5q）；−7；−17/abn（17p） Complex karyotype，monosomal karyotype Wild-type *NPM1* and *FLT3-ITD*^{high} Mutated *RUNX1* Mutated *ASXL1* Mutated *TP53*

注：[*].NCCN 指南 2022.V3。

附录2 CML 在 TKI 治疗后的疗效反应[*]

BCR/ABL（IS）	治疗时间			
	3个月	6个月	12个月	>12个月
>10%	TKI 可能耐药	TKI 耐药		
>1%~10%	TKI 敏感		TKI 可能耐药	TKI 耐药
≤1%	TKI 敏感			

注：[*].NCCN-CML 指南 2023.V1。

附录3 MDS 的国际预后积分系统（IPSS）

预后变量	积分				
	0	0.5	1	1.5	2
骨髓原始细胞/%	<5	5~10		11~20	21~30
染色体核型 [a]	好	中等	差		
血细胞减少系列 [b]	0~1	2~3			

注：a.预后好核型：正常，-Y, del(5q), del(20q); 预后中等核型：其余异常；预后差核型：复杂（≥3个异常）或7号染色体异常。

b.中性粒细胞绝对计数<$1.8×10^9$/L, Hb<100g/L, PLT<$100×10^9$/L。IPSS 危险度分类：低危，0分；中危-1，0.5~1分；中危-2，1.5~2分；高危，≥2.5分。

附录4 MDS修订国际预后积分系统(IPSS-R)

预后变量	积分						
	0	0.5	1	1.5	2	3	4
细胞遗传学	极好		好			差	极差
骨髓原始细胞/%	≤2		>2~<5		5~10	>10	
血红蛋白/(g·L^{-1})	≥100		80~<100	<80			
血小板计数/×10^9/L	≥100	50~<100	<50				
中性粒细胞绝对计数/×10^9/L	≥0.8	<0.8					

注:极好,-Y.del(llq);好,正常核,del(5q).del(12p).del(20q).del(5q)附加另一种异常;中等,del(7q),+8,+19,i(I7q),其他1个或2个独立克隆的染色体异常;差,-7,inv(3)/t(3q)/del(3q),-7/del(7q)附加另一种异常,复杂异常(3个);极差,复杂异常(>3个)。IPSS-R危险度分类:极低危,≤1.5分;低危,>1.5~3分;中危,>3~4.5分;高危,>4.5~6分;极高危,>6分。

附录 5　MDS 的 WHO 分型预后积分系统（WPSS）

预后变量	积分			
	0	1	2	3
WHO 分类	RCUD、RARS、伴有单纯 del（5q）的 MDS	RCMD	RAEB-1	RAEB-2
染色体核型 [a]	好	中等	差	-
严重贫血 [b]	无	有		

注：RCUD. 难治性血细胞减少伴单系发育异常；RARS. 难治性贫血伴有环状铁粒幼红细胞增多；RCMD. 难治性血细胞减少伴有多系发育异常；RAEB. 难治性贫血伴有原始细胞增多。a. 预后良好核型：正常，-Y，del（5q），del（20q）；预后中等核型：其余异常；预后差核型：复杂（≥3 个异常）或 7 号染色体异常。b. 男性患者血红蛋白<90g/L，女性患者血红蛋白<80g/L。WPSS 危险度分类：极低危，0 分；低危，1 分；中危，2 分；高危，3~4 分；极高危，5~6 分。

附录 6　异基因造血干细胞移植前患者应符合的条件

患者年龄 / 岁	0~65
患者体重 /IBW/%	95%~145%
心脏（EF 值）	≥ 45%
肺（肺功能）	
用力肺活量	≥ 60%
弥散功能	≥ 60%
肝功能	
ALT	≤ 正常值上限的 2 倍
AST	≤ 正常值上限的 2 倍
Tbil	≤ 2mg/dL
肾功能	
血肌酐	≤ 1.5mg/dL
一般情况（Kanofsky 积分）	≥ 60%

附录 7 造血干细胞移植合并症指数（HSCT-CI）

合并症	具体疾病	积分 / 分
心律失常	心房颤动*	1
	心房扑动*	
	病态窦房结综合征*	
	室性心律失常*	
心血管	冠状动脉粥样硬化性心脏病*	1
	充血性心力衰竭*	
	心肌梗死*	
	射血分数<50%§	
炎症性肠病	克罗恩病*	1
	溃疡性结肠炎*	
糖尿病	需要胰岛素和/或口服降糖药治疗*	1
脑血管疾病	一过性脑缺血（TIA）*	1
	缺血性或出血性卒中*	
心理异常	需要心理咨询和/或特殊治疗§	1

造血干细胞移植合并症指数（HSCT-CI）（续）

合并症	具体疾病	积分/分
肝脏疾病，轻度	慢性肝炎 §	1
	胆红素：>ULN，但<1.5×ULN §	
	AST/ALT：>ULN，但<2.5×ULN §	
肥胖	BMI≥35kg/m² （成人）§	1
	BMI≥该年龄95%上百分位数（儿童）§	
感染	预处理前需要持续抗生素治疗 §	1
风湿免疫性疾病	需要治疗 *	2
消化性溃疡	内镜证实且需要治疗 *	2
肾病，中重度	血肌酐>2mg/dl（177μmol/l）§	2
	需要血液透析 §	
	前期肾移植 *	
肺脏疾病，中度	血红蛋白纠正的 DLco 66%~80% 预计值 §	2
	FEV$_1$ 66%~80% 预计值 §	
肺脏疾病，重度	血红蛋白纠正的 DLco≤65% 预计值 §	3
	FEV$_1$≤65% 预计值 §	

造血干细胞移植合并症指数（HSCT-CI）（续）

合并症	具体疾病	积分/分
心脏瓣膜病	无症状的二尖瓣脱垂除外 §	3
前期实体肿瘤	需要手术、化疗和/或放疗（非黑色素瘤的皮肤肿瘤除外）*	3
肝病，重度	肝硬化 § 胆红素>1.5×ULN § AST/ALT>2.5×ULN §	3
		总分：

注：*.在患者既往的任何时间诊断；§.取预处理开始前最近的一次检验值或疾病情况。ULN.正常值上限；DLco.一氧化碳弥散率；FEV_1.一秒用力呼气容积；AST.天冬氨酸转氨酶；ALT.丙氨酸转氨酶；BMI.体重指数。危险分级（总分）：低危，0分；中危，1~2分；高危，3分及以上。血红蛋白校正 DLco=DLco/[Hb（g/dl）×0.069 65]。

附录 8　改良的急性 GVHD Glucksberg 分级

	累及器官		
	皮肤	肝脏 - 胆红素血症 / ($mg \cdot dl^{-1}$)	胃肠道
分期			
1	皮疹面积<25%[a]	2~3 [b]	腹泻量>500ml/d[c] 或持续性恶心 [d]
2	皮疹面积 25%~50%	3~6	腹泻量>1 000ml/d
3	皮疹面积>50%，全身红斑	6~15	腹泻量>1 500ml/d
4	全身红皮病伴大疱形成	>15	严重腹痛和 / 或肠梗阻
分度 [e]			
I	分期 1~2	无	无
II	分期 1~3	分期 1	分期 1

改良的急性 GVHD Glucksberg 分级（续）

	累及器官		
	皮肤	肝脏 - 胆红素血症 / (mg · dl^{-1})	胃肠道
Ⅲ		分期 2~3	分期 2~4
Ⅳ[f]	分期 4	分期 4	

注：a. 使用 9 分法或烧伤图表确定皮疹程度。

b. 以总胆红素表示范围。如果已经记录了导致胆红素升高的其他原因，则将其降 1 级。

c. 腹泻量适用于成人。对于儿童患者，腹泻的量应基于体表面积。如果记录了腹泻的另一个原因，则将其降 1 级。

d. 持续恶心并有胃或十二指肠 GVHD 的组织学证据。

e. 作为授予该等级所需的最低器官受累程度的分级标准。

f. Ⅳ度也可能包括较少的器官受累，但功能状态极度下降。

附录 9　IBMTR 的急性 GVHD 严重度指数

严重度指数	累及皮肤		累及肝脏		累及胃肠道	
	最高分期	皮疹面积	最高分期	胆红素 / ($\mu mol \cdot L^{-1}$)	最高分期	腹泻量 / ($ml \cdot d^{-1}$)
A	1	<25%	0	<34	0	<500
B	2	25%~50%	1~2	34~102	1~2	500~1 500
C	3	>50%	3	103~255	3	>1 500
D	4	水疱	4	>255	4	严重腹痛和肠梗阻

注：基于受累器官最高级别赋予严重指数。

附录10　MAGIC分级标准（aGVHD国际联盟GVHD分度）

分期	皮疹（仅活动性红斑）	肝脏（胆红素，mg/dL）	上消化道	下消化道（排便次数）
0	无活动性（红斑）GVHD皮疹	<2	无或间歇性恶心、呕吐或厌食	成人：<500ml/d或<3次/d 儿童：<10ml/（kg·d）或<4次/d
1	<25%	2~3	持续性恶心、呕吐或厌食	成人：500~999ml/d或3~4次/d 儿童：10~19.9ml/（kg·d）或4~6次/d
2	25%~50%	3.1~6		成人：1 000~1 500ml/d或5~7次/d 儿童：20~30ml/（kg·d）或7~10次/d
3	>50%	6.1~15		成人：>1 500ml/d或>7次/d 儿童：>30ml/（kg·d）或>10次/d

MAGIC 分级标准（aGVHD 国际联盟 GVHD 分度）（续）

分期	皮疹（仅活动性红斑）	肝脏（胆红素，mg/dL）	上消化道	下消化道（排便次数）
4	全身红斑（>50%）伴水疱形成和表皮剥脱（>5%）	>15		严重腹痛伴或不伴肠梗阻或便血（无论排便量如何）

注：整体临床分级（基于最严重的靶器官受累）。

0 度：无任何器官 1~4 期。

Ⅰ度：1~2 期皮肤，无肝脏、上消化道或下消化道受累。

Ⅱ度：3 期皮疹和/或 1 期肝脏和/或 1 期上消化道和/或 1 期下消化道。

Ⅲ度：2~3 期肝脏和/或 2~3 期下消化道，0~3 期皮肤和/或 0~1 期上消化道。

Ⅳ度：4 期皮肤、肝脏或下消化道受累，0~1 期上消化道受累。

附录 11　慢性移植物抗宿主病的临床征象

受累器官或者部位	诊断性征象（诊断充分）	区分性征象（诊断不充分）	共同征象（急慢性 GVHD 可见）
皮肤	皮肤异色病、扁平苔藓样变、硬皮病	色素脱失	红斑、斑丘疹
指甲		病甲、甲软化、甲脱离	
头发和体毛		脱发、斑秃	
口腔	扁平苔藓样变，口腔活动受限	口干、黏液囊肿、溃疡、假膜	牙龈炎、黏膜炎、红斑
眼		角膜结膜炎、Sicca 综合征（泪腺功能障碍）	
生殖系统	扁平苔藓样，阴道/尿道挛缩	糜烂、龟裂、溃疡	

慢性移植物抗宿主病的临床征象(续)

受累器官或者部位	诊断性征象（诊断充分）	区分性征象（诊断不充分）	共同征象（急慢性 GVHD 可见）
消化道	食管网格形成，狭窄或硬化		厌食、恶心、腹泻
肝脏			混合性肝炎
肺	活检证实的支气管闭塞	经肺功能或影像学诊断的支气管闭塞	
肌肉、筋膜	筋膜炎、关节挛缩	肌炎和多发性肌炎	
造血系统			血小板减少、嗜酸性粒细胞增多、低或高丙种球蛋白血症、自身抗体形成
其他			心包积液、胸腔积液、腹水

附录 12 慢性移植物抗宿主病（cGVHD）分级评分系统

	0 分	1 分	2 分	3 分
功能评分： □ KPS □ ECOG □ LPS	□无症状，活动完全不受限（ECOG 0；KPS 或 LPS 100%）	□有症状，体力活动轻度受限（ECOG 1；KPS 或 LPS 80%~90%）	□有症状，可自理，<50%时间卧床（ECOG 2；KPS 或 LPS 60%~70%）	□有症状，生活自理受限，>50%时间卧床（ECOG 3~4；KPS 或 LPS<60%）
皮肤、毛发、指甲 □斑丘疹扁平苔藓样变 □丘疹鳞屑样病变或鳞癣 □色素沉着□毛周角化 □红斑□红皮病 □皮肤异色病□硬化改变 □瘙痒症□毛发受累 □指甲受累	□无体表受累 □皮肤无硬化病变	□<18% 体表面积	□19%~50% 体表面积 □皮肤浅层硬化，未绷紧，可捏动	□>50% 体表面积 □皮肤深层硬化 □皮肤绷紧，不可捏 □皮肤活动受限 □皮肤溃疡

慢性移植物抗宿主病（cGVHD）分级评分系统（续）

	0分	1分	2分	3分
□口腔 □有□无扁平苔藓样变	□无症状	□轻度症状，摄入不受限	□中度症状，摄入轻度受限	□严重症状，摄入明显受限
眼睛 □有□无干燥性结膜炎	□无症状	□轻度干眼症（需要滴眼液<3次/d或无症状性干燥性角结膜炎）	□中度干眼症（滴眼液≥3次/d），不伴有视力受损	□严重干眼症，无法工作，视力丧失
胃肠道 □食管狭窄□吞咽困难 □恶心□呕吐□腹痛腹泻 □体重下降	□无症状	□有症状，三个月内体重减轻<5%	□中到重度症状，体重减轻5%~15%，或中度腹泻，不妨碍日常生活	□体重减轻>15%，需要营养支持或食管扩张

慢性移植物抗宿主病（cGVHD）分级评分系统（续）

	0分	1分	2分	3分
肝脏	□总胆红素正常，ALT或碱性磷酸酶<3倍正常值上限	□总胆红素正常，ALT在正常值上限3~5倍，或碱性磷酸酶>3倍正常值上限	□总胆红素升高，但<3mg/dl（51.3μmol/L）或ALT>5倍上限	□总胆红素>3mg/d（51.3μmol/L）
肺	□无症状 FEV$_1$≥80%	□轻度症状（爬1楼气短）FEV$_1$ 60%~79%	□中度症状（平地活动气短）FEV$_1$ 40%~59%	□重度症状（静息气短，需吸氧）FEV$_1$≤39%
关节和筋膜	□无症状	□肢体轻微僵直，不影响日常生活	□四肢至少1个关节僵硬，关节挛缩重度受限	□挛缩伴严重活动受限（不能系鞋带、系纽扣、穿衣等）

慢性移植物抗宿主病（cGVHD）分级评分系统（续）

	0分	1分	2分	3分
生殖系统	□无症状	□轻度症状，查体时无明显不适	□中度症状，检查时轻度不适	□严重症状
总体GVHD严重程度	□非GVHD	□轻度 1个或2个器官受累，得分不超过1分，肺0分	□中度 3个或多个器官受累，得分不超过1分 或者至少有1个器官（不包括肺），得分为2分或者肺1分	□重度 至少有1个器官，得分为3分 或肺评分为2分或3分

附录 13　HSCT 患者 HBV 感染 / 再激活定义

病毒学结果	定义
HBV 原发感染	HBV 阴性患者移植后 HBsAg 阳性和 / 或 HBV-DNA 阳性
HBV 再激活 　慢性 HBV 感染 　既往 HBV 感染	HBV-DNA 比基线升高 ≥ 2log（100 倍），或既往 HBV-DNA- 者 HBV-DNA 升高 ≥ 3log（1 000）IU/ml，或无基线 HBV-DNA 结果者 HBV-DNA 升高 ≥ 4log（10 000）IU/ml HBV-DNA 转阳，HBsAg 转阳

附录 14　乙肝血清免疫学标志物检测内容和临床意义

检测项目	名称	临床意义
HBsAg	乙肝病毒表面抗原	阳性提示被 HBV 感染过或现正在感染者
抗-HBs	乙肝病毒表面抗体	为保护性抗体,其阳性表示对 HBV 有免疫力,见于乙型肝炎康复及接种乙型肝炎疫苗者
HBeAg	乙肝病毒 e 抗原	阳性提示有传染性,往往是乙型肝炎早期或活动期的表现
抗-HBe	乙肝病毒 e 抗体	阳性提示乙肝病毒复制停止或缓慢
抗-HBc	乙肝病毒核心抗体	感染过 HBV 者,无论病毒是否被清除,此抗体多为阳性

附录 15　CMV 感染 / 再激活的诊断

感染类型	诊断标准
原发 CMV 感染	无 CMV 感染史患者检测到 CMV 抗原包括核酸或抗体
再激活的 CMV 血症	有 CMV 感染史（CMV-IgG 阳性）患者外周血检测到 CMV 抗原包括核酸
CMV 相关疾病	
CMV 综合征	在 CMV 血症的基础上出现发热、乏力、肌痛、关节痛等表现，伴有或不伴有 BM 抑制，排除其他原因引起的发热且无 CMV 终末器官疾病
CMV 肺炎	确诊：①出现呼吸困难、低氧血症、肺部间质性改变等症状或体征；②肺活检组织中检测到 CMV 核酸 临床诊断：①出现呼吸困难、低氧血症、肺部间质性改变等症状或体征；② BLAF 中检测到 CMV 拟诊：①出现呼吸困难、低氧血症、肺部间质性改变等症状或体征；②肺活检组织中经 qPCR 检测到 CMV

CMV 感染/再激活的诊断（续）

感染类型	诊断标准
CMV 胃肠炎	确诊：①上消化道或下消化道的症状或体征；②内镜下肉眼可见的黏膜损伤；③消化道黏膜活检组织中检测到 CMV 核酸 临床诊断：①上消化道或下消化道的症状或体征；②消化道黏膜活检组织中检测到 CMV 核酸 拟诊：①上消化道或下消化道的症状或体征；②外周血或活检组织中经 qPCR 检测到 CMV
CMV 视网膜炎	确诊：经眼科专家判定具有典型的相关症状和体征
CMV 脑炎	确诊：①中枢神经系统（CNS）症状和体征；② CNS 活检组织中检测到 CMV 临床诊断：① CNS 症状和体征；② CSF 中检测到 CMV；③影像学或脑电图异常

CMV 感染 / 再激活的诊断（续）

感染类型	诊断标准
CMV 肝炎、肾炎、膀胱炎、心肌炎、胰腺炎及其他终末器官疾病	均只有一个诊断等级，确诊：①相关累及器官的症状和体征；②相应活检组织中检测到 CMV

注：CMV 为双链 DNA 病毒，属于疱疹病毒科 β 亚科，其宿主具有种属特异性，感染人类的 CMV 也称人巨细胞病毒（HCMV）。HSCT 患者的 CMV 感染 / 再激活发生率可达 80%，可引起 CMV 综合征直至器官累及的系列相关性疾病，具有高的病死率。如果不进行 CMV 预防或抢先治疗，CMV 相关疾病的发生率可高达 10%~40%；尽管预防或抢先治疗已经得到广泛应用，仍有 2%~17% 的患者发生 CMV 疾病。近年一些研究结果提示：外周血与组织标本 CMV 存在分离现象，即外周血阴性而组织标本为阳性，这种情况在 CMV 肠炎中尤为常见。

附录 16　CMV 感染 / 再激活的危险因素

移植 0~29d	30~100d	>100d
CMV 感染和终末器官疾病的总体危险因素 - CMV 血清学阳性患者 - 高龄 - 移植类型（非血缘移植、单倍型移植及脐血移植） - 预处理方案（氟达拉滨、抗胸腺细胞球蛋白、阿仑单抗、TBI） **CMV 感染的临床表现** - CMV 血症 - CMV 综合征 - CMV 终末器官疾病在本阶段很少见	**CMV 感染和终末器官疾病的危险因素** 前述危险因素 + - GVHD - T 细胞重建延迟 **CMV 感染的临床表现** - CMV 感染在高危患者中非常常见 - CMV 血症 - CMV 综合征 - CMV 肺炎，该阶段最常见的终末器官疾病 - CMV 胃肠炎	**CMV 感染和终末器官疾病的危险因素** 前述危险因素 + - GVHD - T 细胞重建延迟 **CMV 感染的临床表现** - CMV 感染在高危患者中非常常见 - CMV 血症 - CMV 综合征 - CMV 肺炎，该阶段最常见的终末器官疾病 - CMV 胃肠炎

附录 17 CMV 感染治疗的常用药物及用法

药物	抢先治疗		CMV 疾病	
	剂量	疗程	剂量	疗程
更昔洛韦	5mg/kg b.i.d.	≥2 周(诱导)	5mg/kg b.i.d.	>3 周(诱导)
	5~6mg/kg q.d.	维持治疗直至 CMV 转阴	5~6mg/kg q.d.	维持治疗可考虑
缬更昔洛韦	900mg b.i.d.	≥2 周(诱导)	900mg b.i.d.	>3 周(诱导)
		维持治疗无数据		维持治疗无数据
膦甲酸钠	60mg/kg b.i.d.	≥2 周(诱导)	60mg/kg b.i.d.	>3 周(诱导)
	90mg/kg q.d.	维持治疗直至 CMV 转阴	60mg/kg b.i.d. 或 90mg/kg q.d.	可以考虑维持治疗
西多福韦 [a]	5mg/(kg·周)	至少 3 剂	5mg/(kg·周)	至少 3 剂
	3~5mg/(kg·2 周)	维持治疗直至 CMV 转阴	3~5mg/(kg·2 周)	维持治疗直至 CMV 转阴

注:a. 使用西多福韦时,应予丙磺舒解救。

附录 18 EBV 疾病的诊断

感染类型	诊断标准
原发 EBV 感染	无 EBV 感染史患者检测到 EBV 核酸或抗体
再激活的 EBV 血症	有 EBV 感染史（EBV-IgG 阳性）患者外周血检测到 EBV-DNA
EBV 相关疾病	
EBV 血症伴发热	EBV 血症伴不明原因发热，无明确器官累及。又称 EB 病毒综合征
EBV-PTLD	确诊：①出现累及器官相应症状或体征；②具有相应的组织病理学特征；③组织活检标本中发现 EBV 核酸或编码蛋白 临床诊断（针对未活检患者）：①淋巴结肿大、肝脾大或其他终末器官累及临床表现，排除其他可能的原因；② EBV-DNA 血症
EBV 终末器官疾病	①累及器官出现相应症状/体征；②累及器官活检或分泌物发现 EBV；③排除其他的原因

注：EB 病毒（Epstein-Barr virus, EBV）属 γ 疱疹病毒亚型，90% 以上的成人曾经感染过 EBV，多为隐性感染。感染后 EBV 长期潜伏于 B 淋巴细胞内，当免疫功能低下时可出现 EBV 再激活，导致发热、肺炎、脑炎、肝炎等一系列疾病，在移植包括 HSCT 患者中可引起移植后淋巴细胞增殖性疾病（PTLD）。80%~90% 的 PTLD 为 EBV 阳性 B 淋巴细胞来源，少数为 T 细胞或 NK 细胞来源。根据 WHO 分型，PTLD 分为 4 类：①非破坏性 PTLD；②多形性 PTLD；③单形性 PTLD（包括 B、T 细胞淋巴瘤）；④经典霍奇金淋巴瘤型 PTLD。

附录 19　特异性器官的长期随访评估

	+6 个月	+1 年	每年	说明
眼部				
● 临床正常评估	1	1	1	当出现眼部症状时随时进行
● 视力和眼底检查	+	1	+	关注干燥综合征
预防和保护口腔、牙齿	1	1	1	戒烟 口腔 cGHVD 是发生口腔癌的高危因素,应每半年检查
● 临床评估	1	1	1	
● 牙齿检查	+	1	1	

特异性器官的长期随访评估（续）

	+6 个月	+1 年	每年	说明
呼吸系统				
● 临床评估	1	1	1	cGVHD 患者应进行肺功能检查
● 戒烟	1	1	1	
● 有症状时影像学检查	+	+	+	
心血管系统				
● 心血管疾病危险因素评估	+	1	1	主动控制危险因素
肝脏				
● 肝功能评估	+	1	1	HBV 或 HCV 患者监测病毒载量
● 铁蛋白		1	+	当有铁过载时进行 MRI 检查

特异性器官的长期随访评估（续）

	+6 个月	+1 年	每年	说明
肾脏				
• 血压监测	1	1	1	出现高血压应检查原因并控制
• 尿蛋白检查	1	1	1	避免肾毒性药物
• BUN/Scr 检查	1	1	1	
肌肉结缔组织				
• 体能状态	1	1	1	有 cGVHD 风险时，评估关节活动度和皮肤有无硬化
骨骼				
• 骨密度		1	+	运动、补充钙剂和维生素 D 预防骨质疏松和骨折